Primary Pediatric Radiology

Primary Pediatric Radiology

Susan L. Williamson, M.D.
Professor of Radiology and Chief of Pediatric Radiology
University of New Mexico Health Sciences Center
Albuquerque, New Mexico

W.B. SAUNDERS COMPANY
A Harcourt Health Sciences Company
Philadelphia   London   New York   St. Louis   Sydney   Toronto

W.B. SAUNDERS COMPANY

A Harcourt Health Sciences Company

The Curtis Center
Independence Square West
Philadelphia, Pennsylvania 19106

Library of Congress Cataloging-in-Publication Data

Williamson, Susan L.
　　Primary pediatric radiology / Susan Williamson.— 1st ed.
　　　　p. ; cm.
　　ISBN 0-7216-4180-6
　　1. Pediatric radiology. 2. Diagnosis, Radioscopic. 3. Children—Diseases—Diagnosis.
I. Title.
　　[DNLM: 1. Radiography—Child. 2. Radiography—Infant. 3. Ultrasonography—Child.
4. Ultrasonography—Infant. WN 240 W732e 2002]
RJ51.R3 W535 2002
618.92'00757—dc21

2001034482

PRIMARY PEDIATRIC RADIOLOGY　　　　　　　　　　　　　　ISBN 0-7216-4180-6

Printed in the United States of America

Last digit is the print number:　9　8　7　6　5　4　3　2　1

Dedicated to the memory of

JEAN SPIEGEL, M.D.
My co-author, who passed away shortly after we started this book

DENNIS MCALLEN, RT(R)
One of the best pediatric radiographers I have ever known

Preface

Primary Pediatric Radiology provides an introduction to the discipline of pediatric radiology that is particularly suited for pediatric house officers and beginning radiologists. I wanted the book to be helpful not only to radiologists, pediatricians, and family practitioners but also to radiographers, technologists, nurses, and any others who would like more information on pediatric imaging.

I divided the book into two sections: The Neonate (the child up to 28 days of age) and The Older Infant and Child (ages 1 month to 18 years). Although similar, these two groups possess many differences that must be considered when one is viewing radiographs. Each section provides an overview of normal anatomy because the foundation for interpreting abnormal radiologic images rests on a thorough understanding of normal anatomy and its appearance.

Without this basic knowledge, it is impossible to correctly interpret radiographs.

Chapters are based on the clinical presentation of disease. This approach will assist the reader in drawing conclusions and arriving at a correct diagnosis based on the patient's radiographic signs, as opposed to having to know every possible disease before a diagnosis can be made. I feel that this facilitates the learning process and makes for a much more user-friendly text. I have included specific technical considerations and common mistakes, as well as memory hints and charts for quick reference. Also included is a chapter on recognizing cases of child abuse.

I hope that this book creates for the reader the same sense of enthusiasm and enjoyment of pediatric imaging that I have experienced throughout my career as a pediatric radiologist.

Acknowledgments

All authors know that they do not work alone. I would be remiss in not thanking those who have helped me complete this monumental task. I would like to acknowledge the contributions of my colleagues, technologists, and support personnel from the Department of Radiology at the University of New Mexico Health Sciences Center. I would like to recognize Floyd Willard, our staff photographer, who spent a great deal of time preparing images for this book, also, Joseph Tafoya, who completed the task after Mr. Willard's untimely death. Joseph's photographic expertise has been invaluable in the completion of this book. I would also like to thank Charlotte Hendrix of the University of New Mexico Radiology Publishing Office for her valuable contributions in editing and assembling the manuscript. Most of all I would like to thank my husband, Mike Williamson, M.D., and my children for their patience and support throughout this entire process.

Susan L. Williamson

Contents

Introduction

Diagnostic radiology employs many different imaging modalities. A basic book about pediatric radiology should therefore include basic definitions of words commonly used in radiology. These words are grouped according to the various imaging modalities to which they are related.

RADIOGRAPHS

X-ray. Picture generated by passing an x-ray through a body part and onto a film where part of the x-ray is absorbed and part of it is not. The part that is absorbed is white (i.e., bone) and the other is black (i.e., air in lung).

AP (Anteroposterior) View. Radiograph where x-ray beam passes from anterior to posterior body part before it reaches film cassette. Portable x-ray examinations are taken AP; the heart is further from the film and thus is more magnified.

PA (Posteroanterior) View. Radiograph where x-ray beam passes from posterior to anterior body part before it reaches film cassette. Chest x-rays taken in department are PA; heart is closer to film, and thus there is less magnification.

Lateral View. Side view of body parts taken at 90 degrees to frontal view (AP or PA).

Cross-table Lateral. Horizontal beam passes through body part from side.

Decubitus View. Horizontal beam passes through body part that is turned on its right or left side.

ULTRASOUND (US)

US. Image generated by passing ultrasound beam through body part and receiving returning sound depending on density of tissue through which it passes.

Echolucent/Anechoic. Void of internal echoes. Seen with fluid-filled structures (i.e., cyst) and homogenous structures (i.e., lymphomatous lymph nodes). Seen as black on images.

Echogenic/Hyperechoic. Many internal echoes. Seen in structures with many interfaces (i.e., vascular structures). Seen as varying shades ranging from gray to white.

MAGNETIC RESONANCE IMAGING (MRI)

MRI. Image generated by putting body part in magnetic field, which causes protons in the body to align parallel to the field. The protons are given energy or "excited" by an electromagnetic pulse. A signal is generated when the electromagnetic pulse is turned off and the protons return to a steady state. The signal is then converted into an image by a computer.

T1-weighted Image. Best for demonstrating anatomy. All water-filled structures are black and fat structures are white.

T2-weighted Image. Best for demonstrating pathology. Fluids, including pathologic edema, are white.

NUCLEAR MEDICINE

Image generated when radiopharmaceutical, which has been injected, ingested, or inhaled, goes to a specific organ and accumulates there while emitting radiation. The radiation is then collected on a specific camera (gamma camera).

COMPUTED TOMOGRAPHY (CT)

CT. Image generated when an x-ray beam passes through a body in circular fashion. The amount of x-ray that doesn't get absorbed gets detected and the computer generates an image with the data collected from the detectors.

Spiral or Helical CT. A quick CT method that uses continuous scanning in a spiral fashion with a resultant acquisition of a volume of data that can be reconstructed without losing any diagnostic information.

High-resolution CT. A CT method that uses a special reconstruction algorithm to generate an image with better edge detail than the usual reconstruction algorithm used with conventional CT.

Hounsfield Units. Measure of densities on a computerized image. Negative numbers equal fat or air; highly positive numbers equal bone.

The imaging modality used depends on the clinical problem. Specific modalities to use for diagnosis will be emphasized in subsequent chapters.

This book is divided into two sections—The Neonate and The Older Infant and Child—because each age group has unique problems. Each section is then organized according to a problem-oriented approach, similar to the format used by several clinical pediatric texts.

Section I

The Neonate

Chapter 1

The Normal Neonatal Chest

Chest radiography is the chief imaging modality used to evaluate the neonate with respiratory distress. It is one of the most frequently obtained radiographs in this age group. Before the discussion of pathology, an orientation into looking at a chest film is provided.

TECHNICAL FACTORS

Every film should have a "right" or a "left" marker on it. In the neonate, especially, the determination of situs must be ascertained. In addition, the label on the film stating the patient's name should be reviewed to make sure that the correct patient was radiographed.

On an adequately exposed film, the vertebral disc spaces should be seen (Fig. 1–1). The lungs should be able to be evaluated on a view box without the aid of an accessory light or "hot light." Rotation can be easily observed by comparing anterior ribs side-to-side. The degree of rotation of the exam can mislead the observer. For example, the cardiac silhouette can project on the wrong side, mediastinal shift can be simulated when it is not really there, and one hemithorax can appear to be more opaque (Fig. 1–2). Assessing the depth of inspiration is important and can make pathology appear simulated. Eight posterior (horizontal portion) ribs of inflation are average for the neonate. Also, look for cardiac monitor leads and ventilator hoses that might obscure pathology.

EVALUATING CHEST RADIOGRAPHS

Once these technical factors have been assessed, one needs to have a system for looking at the film. Since lung pathology is the most desired observation to be made, it is important to look at other areas first so that these regions are not overlooked. These areas are as follows: bones of the chest, the area under the hemidiaphragm, the cardiomediastinal contour, which includes an evaluation of tubes and lines, and, finally, evaluation of the lung parenchyma.

Thoracic Cage

Evaluation of the bones involves counting the actual number of ribs as well as looking at their morphology. The number of ribs not only can help to assess depth of inflation as already discussed but can also help to diagnose certain syndromes that have unusual rib counts. For example, only 11 rib pairs are common in Down syndrome. Also, the location of umbilical catheters can more accurately be assessed if the actual rib count is obtained. Patients with the VACTERL (V = vertebra, A = anorectal, C = cardiac, TE = tracheoesophageal, R = rib or renal, L = limb) association can have both unusual numbers of ribs and unusual rib deformity. Fractures of ribs can rarely be seen at birth. Patients with trisomy 18 have very thin ribs (Fig. 1–3). Extremely premature infants and some infants with congenital neuromuscular abnormalities can also have thin ribs.

Possible vertebral anomalies can be present such as hemivertebrae (Fig. 1–4) (partial formation of a vertebral body), butterfly vertebrae (midline fusion anomaly of the vertebral body), or block vertebrae (incomplete separation of two or more vertebral bodies). Vertebral anomalies can be associated with underlying renal abnormalities. Sacral anomalies can be associated with anorectal problems.

The shape of the thorax is important. A bell-shaped thorax (Fig. 1–5) is not normal and can be caused by intrinsic hypotonia of the child, maternal sedation, lung hypoplasia, and iatrogenic sedation of the infant.

On the lateral view of the chest, an assessment of the manubrial and sternal ossification centers is important. Usually there is one manubrial ossification center and from two to seven sternal ossification centers (Fig. 1–6). Down syndrome patients frequently have two manubrial ossification centers. Patients with underlying congenital heart disease can have ossification centers with an unusual appearance. Trisomy 18 infants have very small and dysplastic ossification to their sternum and manubrium (Fig. 1–7).

The presence of ossified proximal humeral epiphyseal centers indicates that the infant is term, although the center is not always there at term. Usually it ossifies within the first 3 months. If there is delay in ossification, hypothyroidism may be present.

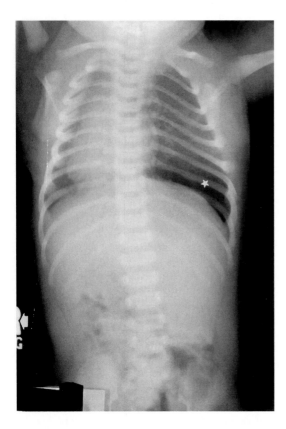

Figure 1–1. Patient with situs inversus totalis (note the arrow indicating "right"). A basilar pneumothorax *(star)* is seen on the patient's left side. If the situs went unrecognized in this patient, the wrong hemithorax could get needle aspiration.

Figure 1–2. Rotated frontal view causing apparent mediastinal shift and projection of umbilical vein catheter to the patient's left *(arrow)*.

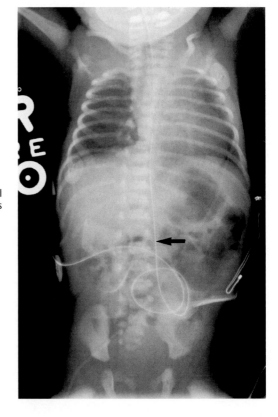

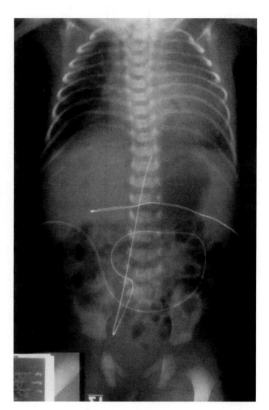

Figure 1–3. Patient with trisomy 18 demonstrating very thin ribs as well as a large cardiac silhouette due to underlying congenital heart disease, which is frequent in these patients.

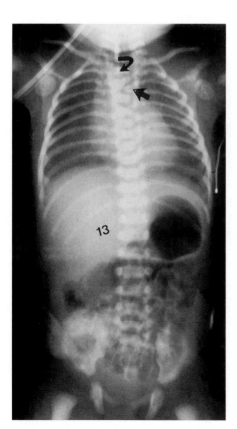

Figure 1–4. Frontal view of patient with VACTERL association including esophageal atresia with orogastric tube in proximal pouch *(curved arrow)* plus tracheoesophageal fistula, vertebral anomalies *(straight arrow)*, and 13 pairs of ribs.

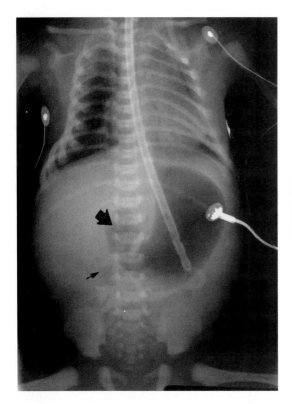

Figure 1–5. Bell-shaped thorax in a patient with Down syndrome. Lungs are clear and the abdomen demonstrates plain film findings of duodenal obstruction with dilated duodenal bulb *(large arrow)* and decompressed gut distally *(small arrow)*.

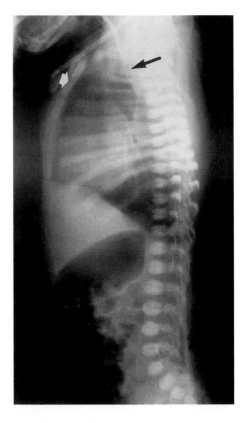

Figure 1–6. Lateral view of patient with VACTERL association and a double manubrial ossification center *(white arrow)*. The enteric tube is stuck in the proximal esophageal pouch *(black arrow)*.

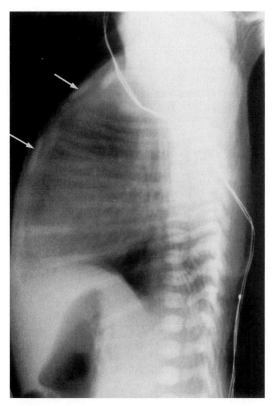

Figure 1–7. Lateral view of patient with trisomy 18 showing hypoplastic sternal and manubrial ossification centers *(arrows)*.

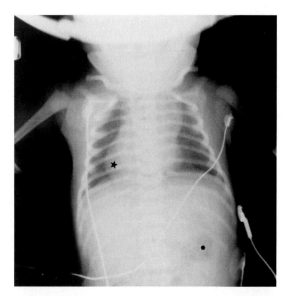

Figure 1–8. Frontal view of patient with severe cyanotic congenital heart disease showing the cardiac apex *(star)* on the side opposite the stomach bubble *(asterisk)*.

Area Under the Hemidiaphragms

The region under the hemidiaphragms is an important location for pathology. Placement of the stomach bubble in an unusual location can lead to a diagnosis of underlying congenital heart disease. For example, if the stomach bubble is on the opposite side from the cardiac apex, the patient has a high incidence of cyanotic congenital heart disease (Fig. 1–8). Midline stomach bubble placement may lead to a diagnosis of not only congenital heart disease but also splenic abnormalities, as seen in the situs ambiguus category. Situs ambiguus is divided into asplenia, which is bilateral right-sidedness, and polysplenia, bilateral left-sidedness.

In addition, the presence or absence of unusual gas collections in the abdomen should be sought. Air in the portal vein is a result of pneumatosis intestinalis, which is the hallmark of necrotizing enterocolitis (Fig. 1–9). Free air in the abdomen may also be present and is diagnosed by seeing abnormal lucency over the liver, creating more than one shade of gray over this structure (Fig. 1–10).

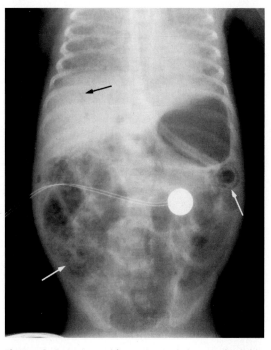

Figure 1–9. Patient with pneumatosis intestinalis *(white arrows)* and portal venous air seen in the liver *(black arrow)*.

Cardiomediastinal Contour

The thymus in a healthy neonate is large, although stress can cause it to atrophy in as little as 24 hours. Because the normal thymus has a soft makeup, it can have a wavy margin

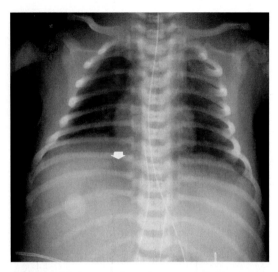

Figure 1–10. Lucency *(arrow)* seen over the liver represents free intraperitoneal air.

caused by the impression of the anterior ribs (Fig. 1–11).

Because the normal thymus in a neonate can cause the appearance of an enlarged heart, the lateral view is essential to distinguish a normal-sized heart with a prominent thymus from that of an enlarged heart. On the lateral view, the heart shadow, where it intersects the hemidiaphragm, should not project behind the inferior vena cava (IVC) shadow, where it intersects the hemidiaphragm (Fig. 1–12).

The side of the aortic arch should be located, although this is difficult in the neonate due to the overlying thymus shadow. Usually the trachea shifts away from the side of the arch and the pedicles of the thoracic spine are denser on the side of the descending aorta, which is usually the same side as the arch (Fig. 1–13A). Occasionally, a right aortic arch can be diagnosed by a high umbilical artery catheter (Fig. 1–13B).

Continuity of the esophagus must be established. This is frequently confirmed by the presence of an orogastric tube extending to the stomach in the patient. If there is no orogastric tube, a lateral view can help to assess continuity. When there is proximal esophageal atresia, there is an air-filled pouch that pushes the trachea anteriorly. If there is a distal tracheoesophageal fistula, there will be air in the stomach and intestine (Fig. 1–4).

Tubes and Lines

Tubes and lines must be evaluated. If an endotracheal tube (ETT) is present, it should reside somewhere between the thoracic inlet and the carina. Care must be made to ascertain that the ETT is really in the trachea and not in the esophagus. A lateral may be necessary to determine tube position accurately (Fig. 1–14). Umbilical vessel catheters that can extend into the thorax are the umbilical artery catheter (UAC) and the umbilical vein catheter (UVC). On a frontal view of the neonate's entire trunk, the UAC is seen to course inferiorly before heading in a cephalad direction. If a lateral view is obtained, the UAC is seen to lie posteriorly against the vertebral bodies since it courses in the aorta. This catheter should be somewhere between the T6 and T9 vertebral bodies or at the L3 vertebral body level. The UVC courses anteriorly and superiorly to the level of the heart. The location of this catheter is above or below the liver but not projecting within the substance of the liver. The ideal location of the UVC is at the junction of the right atrium and IVC (Fig. 1–15).

Lung Parenchyma

Assessment for degree of inflation is important. A normal neonate inflates to around eight posterior ribs. (The posterior ribs are the horizontal portions of the ribs.) Hypoinflation can sometimes result in lung opacities that aren't real. In comparing radiographs, one rib difference in inflation can cause a great deal of difference in the appearance of the lungs. Generally neonates and young children respond to lung pathology by being hyperinflated. The one exception is in a pre-

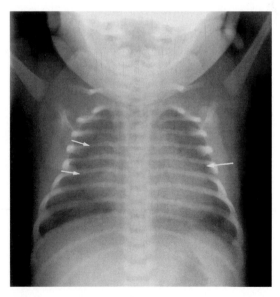

Figure 1–11. Prominent thymus showing a wavy margin bilaterally *(arrows)* due to anterior rib impression.

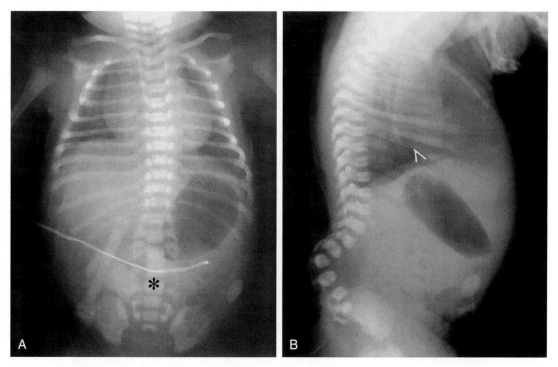

Figure 1–12. A, Frontal view of patient with myelodysplasia *(asterisk)* and a prominent thymus. **B,** The lateral view shows where the heart intersects the hemidiaphragm anterior to the inferior vena cava shadow *(lines)*.

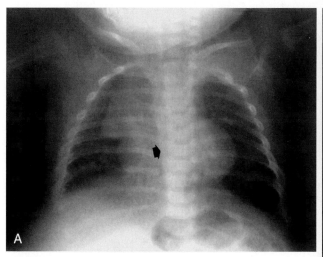

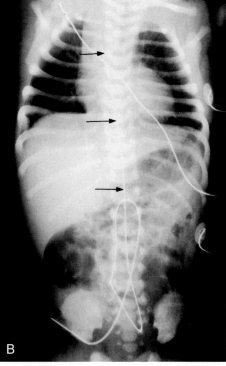

Figure 1–13. A, Frontal view of patient with right aortic arch. Pedicles are dense on the right because of the descending aorta *(arrow)*. **B,** Another patient with a right aortic arch demonstrated by the high umbilical artery catheter *(arrows)*.

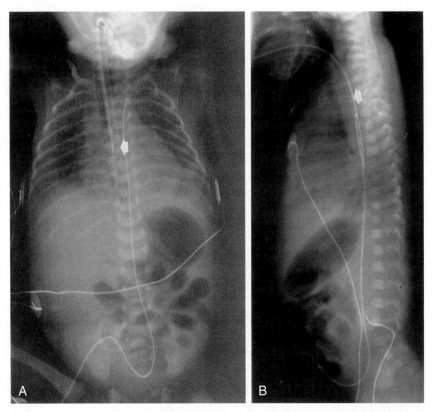

Figure 1–14. A, Patient with endotracheal tube projecting deep *(arrow)*, but the lateral view **(B)** shows that it is in the esophagus *(arrow)*.

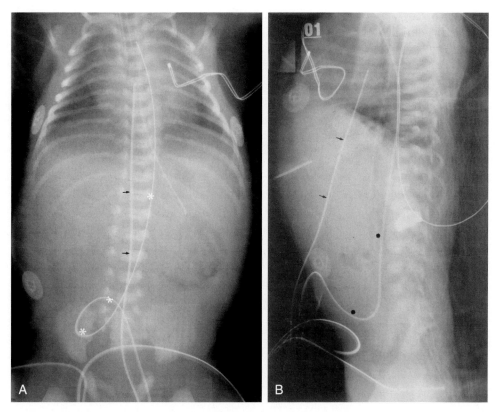

Figure 1–15. A, Frontal view showing umbilical artery catheter (UAC) *(asterisks)* and umbilical vein catheter (UVC) *(arrows)*. The UAC dips inferiorly in the pelvis and projects posteriorly on the lateral view. **B,** The UVC heads straight cephalad on the AP view and is anterior on the lateral view.

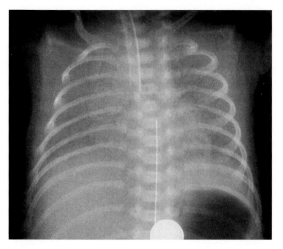

Figure 1–16. Typical fluffy appearance of the alveolar filling process—surfactant deficiency disease in a neonate.

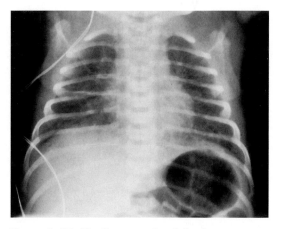

Figure 1–17. The linear streaks of density represent a typical interstitial process seen in this neonate who has transient tachypnea of the newborn.

mature infant with surfactant deficiency in which the lungs are hypoinflated before the patient is mechanically ventilated.

The last step in looking at a chest radiograph is the evaluation of lung parenchyma for pathology. Usually the pathology is divided into alveolar filling processes and interstitial processes. In general, the alveolar processes are fluffy in appearance and the interstitial processes are linear in appearance. Substances that fill up the alveoli such as blood, pus, water, protein, and cells cause the fluffy appearance or a frank "white out" of the lungs as in the neonate with surfactant deficiency disease (Fig. 1–16). The most common interstitial process in the neonate is transient tachypnea of the newborn (Fig. 1–17). Not only does this process cause linear streaks in the lungs but the presence of bronchial wall thickening can also be seen. In the neonate, the differentiation of these processes into interstitial versus alveolar can be difficult.

Chapter 2

The Neonate with Respiratory Distress

Respiratory distress in the neonate is one of the most common clinical problems. The chest radiograph is the diagnostic procedure of choice for evaluation of this entity. Respiratory distress in the neonate can be divided into two categories: medical and surgical. The surgical conditions require surgery to cure the respiratory distress, and the medical ones require medical support such as antibiotics, oxygen, or ventilators in order to achieve a cure (Table 2–1).

The medical causes vary slightly if the neonate is a premature infant and not a term infant. A preemie can suffer from infantile respiratory distress syndrome and immature lung syndrome, whereas a term infant usually does not. The exception is an infant of a diabetic mother, as these infants may have delay in lung maturation. On the other hand, a term infant can have meconium aspiration syndrome, but a preemie will not. Both these groups of infants can suffer from transient tachypnea of the newborn, persistent fetal circulation, and neonatal pneumonia. Unlike the medical conditions, the surgical conditions can affect both premature and term infants. The surgical conditions are made up of masses and masslike condi-

tions as well as airway pathology that require surgical correction.

MEDICAL CAUSES OF RESPIRATORY DISTRESS IN THE NEONATE

Infantile Respiratory Distress Syndrome

Infantile respiratory distress syndrome (IRDS), also known as hyaline membrane disease and surfactant deficiency disease, is the only one of the medical conditions causing respiratory distress that presents with hypoinflation in the patient who is not being mechanically ventilated (Fig. 2–1). The radiographs also show diffuse symmetric opacities, sometimes referred to as "granular" with air bronchograms, extending to the periphery of the lungs. Air bronchograms are sometimes more obvious after the patient has been intubated. (Air bronchograms in the medial one third of the lung are a normal finding.) Asymmetric findings occur when the endotracheal tube (ETT) is deep (Fig. 2–2) or when the surfactant is distributed asymmetrically. Pleural effusions are not part of the picture. When effusions are present, another-

Table 2–1. RESPIRATORY DISTRESS IN THE NEONATE

MEDICAL CAUSES OF RESPIRATORY DISTRESS		SURGICAL CAUSES OF RESPIRATORY DISTRESS	
Preterm	*Term*	*Masses*	*Airway Pathology*
			Tracheoesophageal fistula with or without esophageal atresia
Infantile respiratory distress syndrome	Meconium aspiration	Diaphragmatic hernia	Choanal atresia
Transient tachypnea of the newborn	Pneumonia	Cystic adenomatoid malformation	Bony inlet stenosis
Pneumonia	Transient tachypnea of the newborn	Congenital lobar emphysema	Air leak
Immature lung	Persistent fetal circulation	Sequestration	Hypoplastic lungs
Persistent fetal circulation		Pleural effusion	Innominate artery compression syndrome

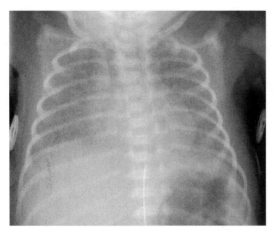

Figure 2–1. Typical changes of infantile respiratory distress syndrome showing hypoinflation in the nonintubated premature lung and a diffuse symmetric granular appearance to the lungs.

diagnosis should be entertained. The radiographic findings of IRDS usually clear rapidly when exogenous surfactant is given.

Complications of IRDS are

- Persistent patent ductus arteriosus (PDA) with left-to-right shunting
- Air leak including pulmonary interstitial emphysema (PIE), pneumomediastinum, pneumothorax, and pneumopericardium
- Pulmonary hemorrhage

The radiographic appearance of PDA and pulmonary hemorrhage are similar in that both can cause a "white out" of the lung parenchyma (Fig. 2–3). If the shunting through the PDA is not that large, the lungs will not be completely opaque and the cardiac silhouette will be visibly larger.

Air leak is usually due to mechanical ventilation. It is seen less commonly now that surfactant is so widely used. The surfactant causes the lungs to be more compliant and allows for the ventilator settings to be lower with resultant less complicating air leak. Pneumothorax causes lucency in the anteromedial and basilar areas of the thorax first due to the supine position of the patient (Fig. 2–4). The costophrenic angle can be especially lucent and sharp with a basilar pneumothorax, which is known as a deep sulcus sign. PIE is due to alveolar rupture into the interstitium of the lungs and causes lucent areas in the lungs that are either circular or linear (Fig. 2–5). Pneumomediastinum causes the air to collect on both sides of the mediastinum and uplifts the thymus shadow (Fig. 2–6). It can dissect into the neck, but more commonly, it dissects into the abdomen. Pneumopericardium causes air to encircle the heart and stops at the base of the heart, that is, at the origin of the great vessels (Fig. 2–7).

Transient Tachypnea of the Newborn

Also known as wet lung and retained fetal lung fluid, transient tachypnea of the newborn (TTN)

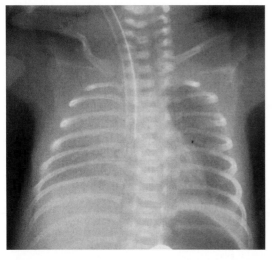

Figure 2–2. Patient with asymmetric lung disease (infantile respiratory distress syndrome) simulating pneumonia because of the deep endotracheal tube (ETT) position. Because the ETT has a beveled end, the right mainstem position actually results in preferrential aeration of the left lung.

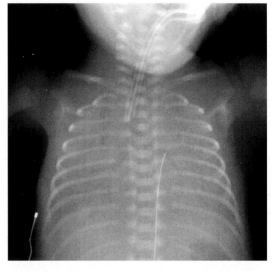

Figure 2–3. Patient with infantile respiratory distress syndrome and a "white out" of the lungs due to pulmonary hemorrhage. Congestive heart failure from patent ductus arteriosus can have similar findings.

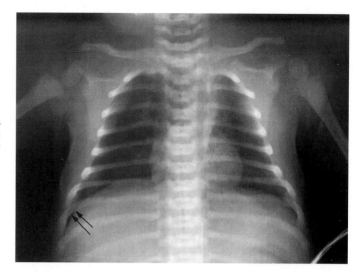

Figure 2–4. Patient with respiratory distress who has a basilar pneumothorax showing the deep sulcus sign *(arrows)* but no evidence of other abnormality.

is the continued presence of fetal lung fluid in the thorax once the infant is born. It is classically seen in neonates that are delivered by cesarean section because they do not experience the thoracic squeeze that vaginal delivery affords. But this condition can also be seen in those infants that are born via vaginal delivery and are simply small in size. The radiographs show hyperinflated lungs in the nonintubated patient with linear, streaky densities throughout and pleural effusions, as well as fluid in the fissures. Pleural fluid is diagnosed in a supine neonate when the edge of the lung laterally, where it normally touches the inner aspect of the rib, is separated by a gray opacity. Fluid in the fissures

results in "lines" in the chest where the fissures normally reside. These radiographic changes clear rapidly, usually in a matter of hours, and certainly within 2-days (Fig. 2–8). Clinically, these patients also get better quickly, and follow-up films are frequently not necessary.

Neonatal Pneumonia

Neonatal pneumonia is bacterial in origin, usually β-hemolytic streptococci. The usual route of transmission of the bacterium is through aspiration of infected secretions. Radiographically, the hallmarks of neonatal pneumonia are hyperin-

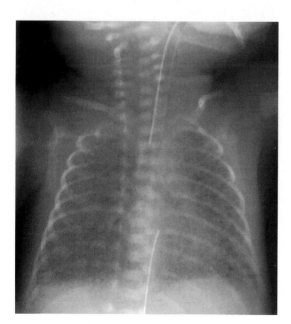

Figure 2–5. Diffuse black lucencies radiating from the hilum to the periphery of the lungs is characteristic of pulmonary interstitial air. The left lung is more involved than the right.

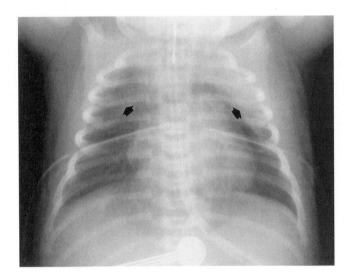

Figure 2–6. Pneumomediastinum is diagnosed by seeing air uplifting the thymus *(arrows)*. Frequently the air can be seen to cross the midline, as in this case.

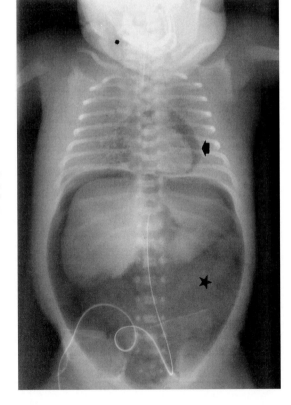

Figure 2–7. Air surrounding the heart and stopping at the base of the heart is pneumopericardium *(arrow)*. Air dissecting into the neck *(asterisk)* and into the abdomen *(star)* from previous pneumomediastinum that is no longer seen on this exam.

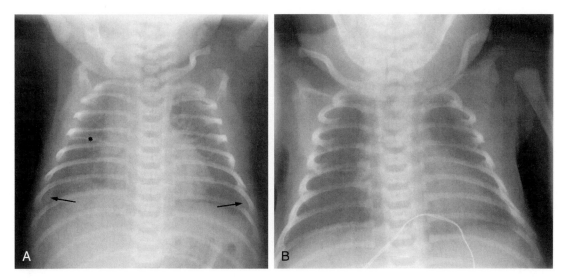

Figure 2–8. A, Transient tachypnea of the newborn (TTN) with fluid seen in the minor fissure *(asterisk),* bilateral pleural effusions *(arrows),* and linear streaky densities. **B,** All these changes improved rapidly in a matter of hours, confirming the diagnosis of TTN.

flated lungs with patchy air space densities and pleural effusion in at least two thirds of the cases (Fig. 2–9). However, neonatal pneumonia can look like anything. Whenever transient tachypnea of the newborn is suspected, neonatal pneumonia should also be considered. The follow-up exam should help distinguish the entities. If there is not considerable improvement in a matter of hours or a day, then pneumonia should be the diagnosis.

Meconium Aspiration Syndrome

Meconium aspiration syndrome occurs when the infant has been stressed in utero for some reason and defecates. The resultant aspiration of me-

conium causes a chemical pneumonitis and non-compliant lungs. As a result, air leak is frequently associated with the aspirated meconium and sometimes there is persistence of pulmonary arterial hypertension (also known as persistent fetal circulation—PFC). If the PFC persists and the patient cannot be oxygenated because of the persistent right-to-left shunting through the PDA and foramen ovale, then the patient is a candidate for extracorporeal membrane oxygenation (ECMO).

Radiographically, the appearance of the chest radiograph in a patient with meconium aspiration syndrome is one of hyperinflation with patchy air space densities throughout (Fig. 2–10A). Distinguishing this entity from neonatal pneumonia is

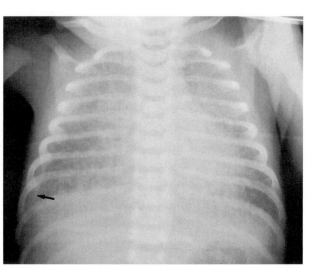

Figure 2–9. The lungs are hyperinflated and show a diffuse alveolar filling process and a right-sided pleural effusion *(arrow).* All these findings are consistent with neonatal pneumonia.

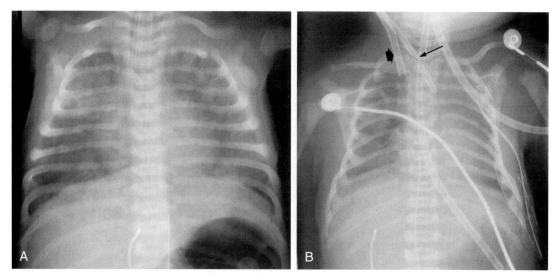

Figure 2–10. A, Patient with meconium aspiration syndrome with diffuse patchy air space densities, indistinguishable from neonatal pneumonia. **B,** Patient on extracorporeal membrane oxygenation (ECMO) with a cannula in the venous system *(wide arrow)* and one in the arterial *(thin arrow)* system, so-called venoarterial ECMO.

nearly impossible. Pleural effusion is present in only 10 percent of patients with meconium aspiration syndrome. Pneumothorax is present in 25 percent of patients. If the patient needs ECMO (Fig. 2–10*B*), the radiographs frequently become airless while on the machine. As the lungs heal and the pulmonary arterial hypertension decreases, the lungs are gradually inflated and the patient is weaned off ECMO.

Persistent Fetal Circulation

Persistent fetal circulation (PFC) can be associated with the entities previously discussed, but it can also occur by itself. Radiographically, the lungs look almost too clear if there is no underlying cause for PFC. The reason for the increased lucency to the lungs is because there is shunting of blood away from the pulmonary circulation. If the persistent pulmonary hypertension cannot be reversed medically, then the patient may be a candidate for ECMO.

SURGICAL CAUSES OF RESPIRATORY DISTRESS IN THE NEONATE

Masses or Masslike Conditions

Diaphragmatic Hernia. Diaphragmatic hernia can present in the immediate neonatal period with the patient experiencing severe respiratory distress. It can also present later, usually without

severe distress. It may be found because of an abnormal physical finding such as displaced heart sounds. Hernias that present early are large defects that have been present since early in utero. About 90 percent of the time, they are on the left with bowel present in the chest. If the defects are large enough, the stomach and liver are in the chest as well. The abdomen is scaphoid in appearance. The cause of respiratory distress is due to lung hypoplasia. Ipsilateral hypoplasia is due to the mass affect of the hernia contents inhibiting lung development. Contralateral hypoplasia is due to mediastinal shift from the hernia that inhibits lung development on that side, as well.

Radiographically, the air-filled loops of bowel are seen above the expected location of the hemidiaphragm (Fig. 2–11). If the stomach is involved, the orogastric tube projects above the hemidiaphragm. When the defect is right-sided, the liver is usually the structure that is up in the chest (Fig. 2–12). If the diagnosis has been made on a prenatal ultrasound, intubation and orogastric tube decompression happen so quickly that sometimes no air reaches the bowel and the hernia contents have the appearance of a solid, airless mass in the chest. If necessary, ultrasound can be used to confirm the diagnosis.

Cystic Adenomatoid Malformation. A cystic adenomatoid malformation (CAM) is a hamartoma of the lung that has three types. Thus, it can have three different appearances on plain chest

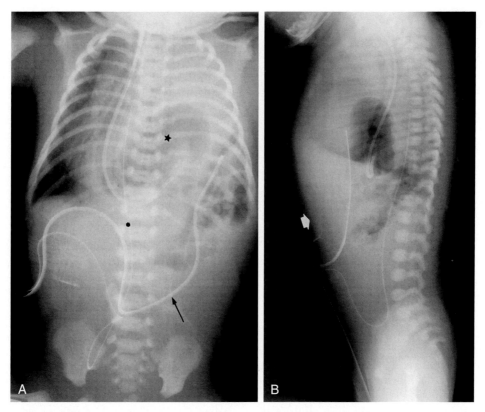

Figure 2–11. Frontal **(A)** and lateral **(B)** views of a patient with a large left-sided diaphragmatic hernia. The umbilical vein catheter *(black arrow)* shows that the liver is in the hernia as well as the stomach *(star)*. The umbilical artery catheter *(asterisk)* is pushed to the patient's right. The abdomen is scaphoid *(white arrow)* on the lateral view.

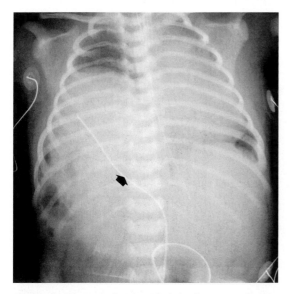

Figure 2–12. Typical right-sided diaphragmatic hernia with liver above the hemidiaphragm. The umbilical vein catheter *(arrow)* helps identify that the liver is above the hemidiaphragm.

radiograph. Type 1 is a mass with a single cyst, type 2 is a mass of multiple cysts, and type 3 is a mass without macrocysts. Usually, the CAM presents as a lobar mass, although the whole lung can be involved. In the neonate's first day of life, the CAM, regardless of type, can look like a solid mass because of delayed clearing of fetal lung fluid from the cystic structure (Fig. 2–13). With time the characteristic appearance is recognized with types 1 and 2. Type 3 retains its solid mass appearance. Before the fetal fluid has cleared, ultrasound can be used to diagnose the fluid-filled cysts. Computerized tomography can also be used in the surgical planning of this entity mainly to localize the process.

Congenital Lobar Emphysema. Congenital lobar emphysema (CLE) is a condition resulting in an obstructed lobe due to bronchial obstruction. It involves only a lobe, most commonly the upper lobes and the middle lobe. It is never in the lower lobes. As with CAM, lobar emphysema is radiographically seen as a solid mass that becomes more hyperlucent once the fetal fluid has

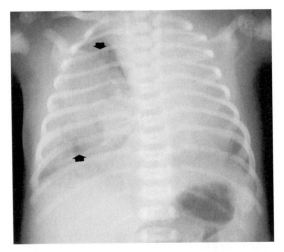

Figure 2–13. Cystic adenomatoid malformation *(arrows)* in right lower lobe is fluid filled immediately after birth and causes a mass effect with shift of the mediastinum to the contralateral side.

cleared (Fig. 2–14). To confirm the diagnosis, a ventilation/perfusion nuclear medicine scan can be done. Using this technique, the perfusion portion of the scan will demonstrate lack of flow to the involved lobe. The ventilation portion will show delayed accumulation of tracer into the involved lobe and then holdup of the tracer in the same lobe.

Lobar Sequestration. Lobar sequestration is pulmonary tissue that has its own arterial blood supply from the systemic arterial system. The pulmonary tissue is nonfunctional but can become superinfected. There are two types: extralobar and intralobar. The extralobar type has its own pleura and is outside the lung. This is the type seen in neonates. The intralobar type is found within the lung and is seen in older patients. On plain film radiography, the sequestration is seen as a mass that is in the left lower lobe about 90 percent of the time. To help confirm the diagnosis, ultrasound can be used to diagnose the systemic arterial blood supply. If the ultrasound is inconclusive, nuclear medicine angiography can be used to confirm the diagnosis. In the past, contrast aortography was performed to diagnose the systemic supply, but this modality is no longer used.

Pleural Effusion. A pleural effusion acts as a mass if it is large enough and causes respiratory distress. The effusion is most often chylous in histologic makeup and is most often on the right. The etiology may be birth trauma but it can be seen more frequently in those patients with Down syndrome. Nonchylous pleural effusions can also be seen with underlying conditions such as sequestrations and pneumonia. On plain chest radiography the effusion presents as a homogeneous opacity that layers posteriorly in the supine neonate (Fig. 2–15). If it is large enough, the entire hemithorax will be opaque, and there will be mediastinal shift to the contralateral side. If the diagnosis is in doubt, ultrasound of the chest can beused to confirm the fluid nature of the opacification.

Airway Pathology

Choanal Atresia. Choanal atresia presents because neonates are obligate nose breathers. If the condition is bilateral, the neonate has no way to

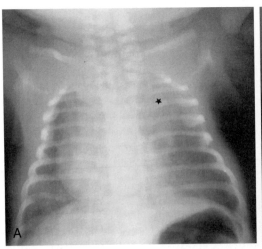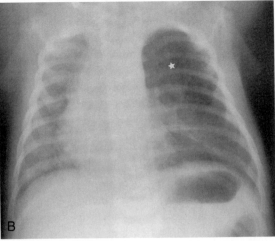

Figure 2–14. A, Left upper lobe congenital lobar emphysema is fluid filled *(black star)* and appears masslike until the fluid is resorbed and the emphysematous appearance *(white star)* results **(B).**

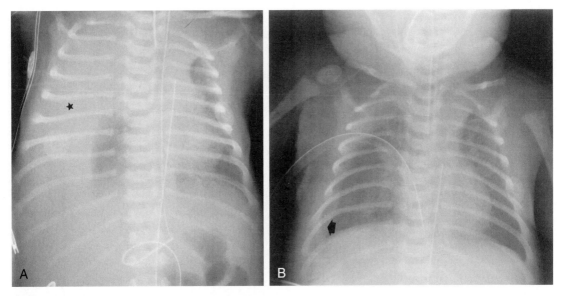

Figure 2–15. A, A large *(star)* chylous right effusion layering posteriorly and causing mediastinal shift to the left. **B,** After chest tube drainage, only a small effusion *(arrow)* can be seen with decreased mediastinal shift.

breathe and is in respiratory distress immediately. The condition can be further suspected by the inability to pass a nasogastric tube through the nose. Confirmation of the diagnosis is made with CT because it best shows the bony abnormality (Fig. 2–16). Before CT became the standard, contrast material was instilled into the nose and plain radiographs were obtained. These showed the blockage but not the anatomic abnormality that was causing the blockage. Choanal stenosis does not cause respiratory distress as severe as does atresia. The CT findings are not as dramatic in

that there is only narrowing of the airway passages with stenosis and not the complete blockage seen with atresia.

Bony Inlet Stenosis. Bony inlet stenosis presents similarly as choanal stenosis, but the site of obstruction is different in that its location is more anterior. Diagnosis is confirmed with CT scanning (Fig. 2–17).

Tracheoesophageal Fistula with or without Esophageal Atresia. Respiratory distress can re-

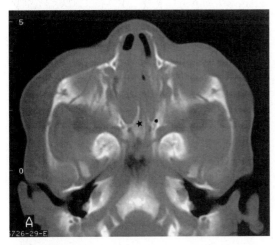

Figure 2–16. Bony changes of choanal atresia with enlargement of the vomer *(star)* and medial bowing of the lateral wall of the nasal cavity *(asterisk).*

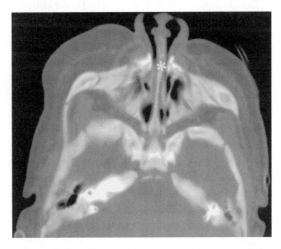

Figure 2–17. Bony inlet stenosis. CT demonstrates marked narrowing of the anterior nasal cavity *(asterisk).*

sult in this entity for two reasons. The first reason being aspiration either through the fistula or from overflow due to the obstructed esophagus and second, tracheomalacia that results from the in utero compression and resultant malformation of the trachea by the dilated and obstructed esophageal pouch. This abnormality is discussed in more detail in Chapter 7.

Air Leak Phenomena. Air leak phenomena, that is, pneumothorax and pneumomediastinum, can occur spontaneously in the newborn when it takes its first breath. As discussed previously, it can also occur with meconium aspiration syndrome, mechanical ventilation, or any cause of noncompliant lungs. Frequently the infant is tachypneic. The pneumothorax may require intervention, especially if there is a tension component to it. This intervention usually involves needling the pneumothorax, followed by a chest tube if the air returns. Diagnosis rests with the plain chest radiograph. Pneumothorax collects first at the bases and anteromedially in the supine infant. When the pneumothorax is large, it is then seen around the periphery of the lung (Fig. 2–18). If the diagnosis of pneumothorax is suspected but cannot be confirmed, a decubitus view with the side in question up can diagnose the condition because the air will collect along the lateral edge of the lung. The diagnosis of tension pneumothorax is made when there is shift of the mediastinum to the contralateral side or depression of the hemidiaphragm, or both. Pneumomediastinum causes the thymus to be uplifted and is present

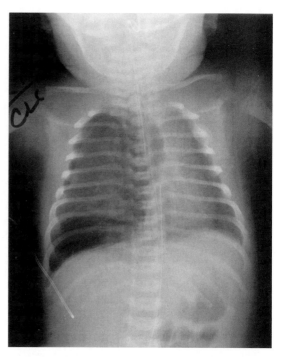

Figure 2–18. Large right-sided pneumothorax with tension as seen by depression of hemidiaphragm and shift of the mediastinum to the left.

on both sides of the mediastinum (Fig. 2–19). Pneumomediastinum rarely needs intervention.

Hypoplastic Lungs. Bilateral hypoplastic lungs is a condition that can cause severe respiratory distress but not much can be done for the condi-

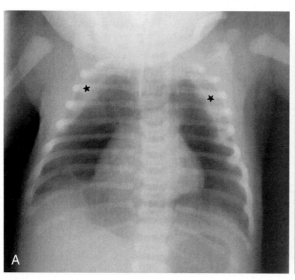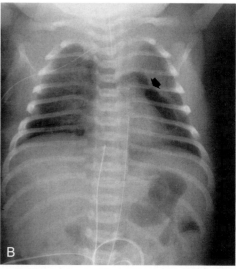

Figure 2–19. A, Large anterior pneumomediastinum causing the lobes of the thymus to be uplifted and plastered against the thoracic cage *(stars).* When the pneumomediastinum is this large, pneumothorax can mistakenly be simulated. **B,** Pneumomediastinum is easier to appreciate when it is smaller *(arrow).*

tion other than supportive care. It is suspected clinically when high ventilator pressures are needed to oxygenate the infant but the radiograph shows small lung volumes (Fig. 2–20). Air leak phenomena frequently occur in association with hypoplastic lungs. A maternal history of oligohydramnios can lead to the diagnosis. It is also seen in some bony dysplasias such as asphyxiating thoracic dystrophy. Diagnosis of hypoplastic lungs can be suspected on the basis of the chest radiograph, which frequently shows the thorax to be bell shaped and the lung volumes to be small subjectively with pneumothorax present.

Unilateral lung hypoplasia can also cause respiratory distress, although not as severe as bilateral involvement. Diagnosis can be suspected when one hemithorax is nearly opaque because the mediastinum has shifted to the opaque side and the ribs remain widely separated (Fig. 2–21). With lung collapse, the ribs are closer together. When lung hypoplasia is present, a cardiac echo needs to be performed to exclude anomalous pulmonary venous return also known as scimitar syndrome or venolobar syndrome.

Innominate Artery Compression Syndrome. This abnormality is caused by a combination of

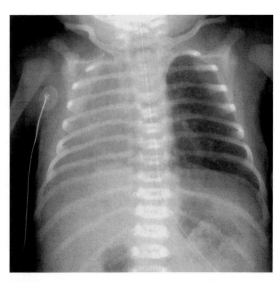

Figure 2–21. Right lung hypoplasia with shift of the mediastinum and maintenance of normal rib separation.

an anomalous origin of the innominate artery from the aortic arch plus a prominent thymus. The artery arises slightly more distally on the arch and causes an anterior tracheal impression as it passes to the right. If the plain film suggests the entity by showing the anterior impression (Fig. 2–22), then MRI can be performed for confirmation. There is an association of this entity in patients with esophageal atresia with or without tracheoesophageal fistula.

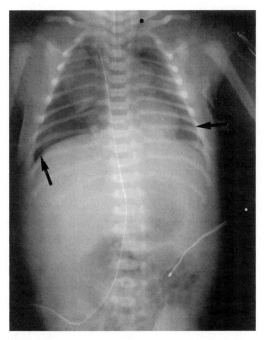

Figure 2–20. Intubated infant with hypoplastic lungs resulting in bilateral pneumothorax *(arrows)* and pneumomediastinum with air dissecting into the neck *(asterisk)*. Umbilical vein catheter projects into superior vena cava.

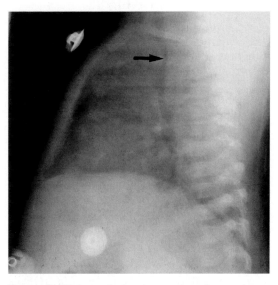

Figure 2–22. Innominate artery compression syndrome is suspected by observing an anterior impression on the trachea at the level of the thoracic inlet *(arrow)*.

Chapter 3

The Neonate with Congestive Heart Failure

Congestive heart failure (CHF) in the neonate does not result from left-to-right shunts such as atrial septal defect, ventricular septal defect, or patent ductus arteriosus unless there is underlying premature lung disease. These lesions do not usually cause difficulty in the neonatal period because the pulmonary vascular resistance is too high to allow for left-to-right shunting to occur at this time. These lesions are discussed later, as they apply to the older infant and child.

Pulmonary venous congestion and congestive heart failure are used interchangeably in this section. The cardiac lesions that cause pulmonary venous congestion in the neonate include left-sided (i.e., left chamber) obstructive lesions, cardiomyopathies, and peripheral arteriovenous malformations. An exception to this gamut is when there is obstruction to pulmonary venous return before it reaches the heart, such as is seen with total anomalous pulmonary venous return below the hemidiaphragm (Table 3–1).

RADIOGRAPHIC FINDINGS

On plain chest radiograph the cardiac silhouette is enlarged and the pulmonary vessels are either normal or indistinct (Fig. 3–1). There may be pleural fluid. However, in the first day of life the chest film is frequently normal. The only exception to this appearance is the patient with obstructed pulmonary veins (Fig. 3–2). The appearance here suggests failure out of proportion to the size of the cardiac silhouette, that is, normal size heart with a failure pattern to the pulmonary vessels. Severe transient tachypnea of the newborn can also resemble this initially.

The lesions in this category causing an enlarged cardiac silhouette cannot be separated on the basis of the chest radiograph. Cardiac echo is the imaging modality of choice.

LEFT-SIDED OBSTRUCTIVE LESIONS

These lesions cause obstruction to the left-sided chambers that result in pulmonary vascular congestion.

Hypoplastic Left Heart Syndrome

Hypoplastic left heart syndrome consists of aortic and mitral valve atresia with an underdeveloped left atrium and left ventricle. The ascending aorta is extremely small and is basically a conduit for retrograde flow from a patent ductus arteriosus into the coronary arteries. It is the most common cause of congestive heart failure in the first week of life. Frequently, there is a normal-appearing chest radiograph in the first day of life. As the pulmonary vascular resistance drops, more pulmonary arterial flow occurs through the right heart, but the pulmonary venous flow can't get out of the heart due to the hypoplastic left chambers. The right heart fails and the cardiac silhouette markedly enlarges as the right-sided chambers enlarge and the pulmonary vascularity becomes indistinct.

Aortic Arch Abnormalities

Aortic arch abnormalities consist of isolated severe coarctation, aortic interruption, hypoplastic aortic arch, and coarctation that also has an intracardiac shunt associated with it, which is known as coarctation syndrome. These aortic arch abnormalities cause a severe pressure overload phenomenon on the left ventricle that causes the left ventricle to fail early. The coarctation syndrome results in both pressure overload and volume overload because of the associated intracardiac shunt. Coarctation of the aorta is also associated with a bicuspid aortic valve in a high percentage of cases, but this valvular lesion usually is not the cause of the patient presenting in the neonatal period.

Critical Aortic Stenosis

Critical aortic stenosis presents in the neonatal period because the valve is markedly hypoplastic and usually consists of one stenotic valve. As a result, the left ventricle is markedly thickened and frequently contracts poorly.

Table 3–1. CONGESTIVE HEART FAILURE IN THE NEONATE

NORMAL-SIZED CARDIAC SILHOUETTE	ENLARGED CARDIAC SILHOUETTE

Obstructed pulmonary veins
   Total anomalous pulmonary venous return obstructed
   Pulmonary vein atresia
   Congenital mitral stenosis
   Cor triatriatum
	Left-sided obstructive lesions
	   Hypoplastic left heart syndrome
	   Aortic arch abnormality
	   Critical aortic stenosis
	Cardiomyopathies
	   Asphyxia
	   Infants of diabetic mothers
	   Arrhythmias
	Peripheral arteriovenous malformations
	   Vein of Galen
	   Hemangioendothelioma

CARDIOMYOPATHIES

Cardiomyopathies result in ventricular dysfunction, which subsequently causes pulmonary vascular congestion.

Asphyxia

Asphyxia is the most common cause of cardiomyopathy in the neonate. The degree of ischemia sustained by the myocardium determines whether or not the cardiac function will get better. Usually when the cardiomyopathy results from asphyxia, other organs are injured as well.

Infants of Diabetic Mothers

Infants of diabetic mothers can have cardiomyopathy that is due to asymmetric septal hypertrophy with accompanying cardiomegaly. This cardiomyopathy is probably due to the hypoglycemia found frequently in these children.

Arrhythmias

Arrhythmias also cause ventricular dysfunction. Paroxysmal atrial tachycardia and complete heart block are two of the arrhythmias that can be seen in the neonate and can cause ventricular dysfunction.

PERIPHERAL ARTERIOVENOUS MALFORMATIONS

Peripheral arteriovenous malformations (AVMs) cause a high output state with eventual ventricular dysfunction and congestive heart failure. The AVMs most commonly encountered are vein of Galen malformations and hemangioendothelioma of the liver. Rare, large AVMs throughout the body can also result in ventricular dysfunction (Fig. 3–3).

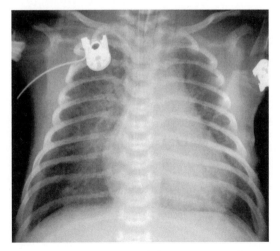

Figure 3–1. Congestive heart failure in a neonate due to a severe left-sided obstructive lesion: coarctation of the aorta.

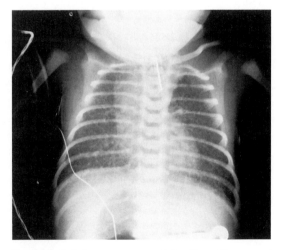

Figure 3–2. Pulmonary venous obstruction with a normal heart size but poor vascular definition in this patient with complex congenital heart disease, including obstructed total anomalous pulmonary venous return.

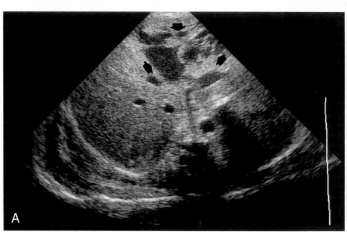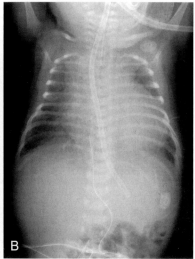

Figure 3–3. A, Arteriovenous malformation involving the left lobe of liver *(arrows)* and resultant high-output congestive heart failure **(B).**

Vein of Galen Malformations

Vein of Galen malformations are found in the head and frequently cause hydrocephalus. Clinically, there is frequently a bruit over the anterior fontanel. Cranial ultrasound is useful in making this diagnosis with the additional use of Doppler, which can detect blood flow.

Hemangioendotheliomas of the Liver

Hemangioendotheliomas of the liver, as discussed in Chapter 6, cause vascular prominence to the liver on ultrasound. These lesions frequently can involute spontaneously (Fig. 6–6).

OBSTRUCTED PULMONARY VENOUS RETURN

Total Anomalous Pulmonary Venous Return Obstructed

Total anomalous pulmonary venous return (TAPVR) obstructed is the most common entity in this category. TAPVR has three main types. Type I is supracardiac with the pulmonary venous drainage occurring into the left vertical vein, then to the left innominate vein, and into the superior vena cava. Type II is intracardiac where the drainage is into the coronary sinus. Type III is infracardiac where the drainage is through a common vein that descends below the hemidiaphragm and usually drains into the liver. Type III TAPVR is always obstructed, and the other two types can be obstructed but not as frequently. Regardless of the type of TAPVR, if it is obstructed, the radiographic finding is the same: failure pattern with a normal-sized cardiac silhouette.

Pulmonary Vein Atresia

This is a rare cause of the same radiographic appearance where no visible pulmonary veins can be identified. This entity is more commonly seen in a unilateral fashion than a bilateral fashion.

Congenital Mitral Stenosis

Acquired mitral stenosis from rheumatic fever is more common than congenital mitral stenosis is. The valve is usually dysplastic and obstructs the pulmonary venous return.

Cor Triatriatum

In this entity the pulmonary veins drain into a chamber behind the left atrium. This chamber then drains into the left atrium through a membrane with a small orifice, which obstructs the pulmonary venous return.

Chapter 4

The Neonate with Cyanosis Due to Congenital Heart Disease

Cyanosis in the patient with congenital heart disease results from either right-to-left shunting through intracardiac shunts or from unoxygenated blood entering the aorta. The first type results in decreased pulmonary blood flow due to an obstruction to the right heart that causes the blood to shunt from the right heart to the left heart. The second type is associated with mixing (admixture lesions or cyanotic shunts) of both oxygenated and unoxygenated blood such that the blood exiting out the aorta is not fully saturated and the patient becomes cyanotic. Because there is mixing, the plain chest radiograph shows increased pulmonary blood flow. The amount of oxygenated blood that mixes with the unoxygenated will determine the level of cyanosis. Usually those patients with right-sided obstruction and decreased pulmonary blood flow are more cyanotic than those with the admixture lesions (Table 4–1).

RADIOGRAPHIC FINDINGS WITH ADMIXTURE LESIONS

In patients with the admixture lesions the radiographic findings are that of an enlarged cardiac silhouette with increased pulmonary vascularity (Fig. 4–1) and a non-border-forming pulmonary outflow tract. In these lesions the pulmonary outflow tract is either not there, as with truncus arteriosus, or is misplaced, as in transposition of the great vessels, so that the pulmonary outflow tract does not form a border. With the usual acyanotic shunts, such as atrial septal defect, patent ductus arteriosus, or ventricular septal defect, the pulmonary outflow tract is in the normal position and is prominent due to the increased amount of pulmonary blood flowing through it (Fig. 4–2). (Remember that patients with acyanotic shunts usually do not present in the neonatal period because the pulmonary vascular resistance is too high.) The pulmonary outflow tract is appropriate for the amount of blood going through it. However, with the cyanotic shunts, the pulmonary outflow tract is not seen and therefore is not considered to be appropriate for the size of the pulmonary vascularity. This radiographic appearance of the cyanotic shunt usually takes a few days to

occur since the thymus tends to atrophy due to stress and the pulmonary vascular resistance needs to drop enough to show the shunt vascularity. These lesions cannot be separated on the basis of the chest radiograph. Cardiac echo is necessary for definitive diagnosis.

Transposition of the Great Vessels

Transposition of the great vessels (TGV) consists of the pulmonary artery arising from the left ventricle and the aorta arising from the right ventricle. Systemic venous return that is unoxygenated then goes out the aorta and the oxygenated pulmonary venous return goes back into the lungs. There would be two entirely separate circulations, except that there is usually some sort of communication between the pulmonary and systemic vascularity such as an atrial septal defect or patent ductus arteriosus. Thus, the admixture component is achieved. If the mixing of blood is not adequate, these patients are candidates for a balloon atrial septostomy in the catheterization laboratory. Eventual repair is usually an arterial switch procedure (Jatene) in appropriate patients. Those patients that are not candidates for the switch procedure will have some sort of atrial baffle procedure to redirect pulmonary venous return to the systemic ventricle (Senning).

Truncus Arteriosus

Truncus arteriosus consists of the pulmonary artery and the aorta being joined together to form a common trunk that rises from both ventricles and usually is associated with a ventricular septal defect. This lesion is associated with a right aortic arch in approximately one third of cases. Truncus arteriosus and all the remaining entities are much less common than TGV.

Single Ventricle

Single ventricle is, as the name implies, a common ventricle from which atria drain and both the aorta and pulmonary artery arise. The mixing of blood occurs in the single ventricle. Repair

Table 4–1. CYANOTIC NEONATE WITH CONGENITAL HEART DISEASE

INCREASED BLOOD FLOW	DECREASED BLOOD FLOW
Admixture lesions (T lesions)	Right-sided obstructive lesions
Transposition of great vessels	Tetralogy of Fallot with pulmonary atresia
Truncus arteriosus	Critical pulmonary valve stenosis
Single (tingle) ventricle	Pulmonary valve atresia with intact ventricular septum
Total anomalous pulmonary venus return unobstructed	Tricuspid atresia
Tricuspid atresia	Ebstein anomaly
Double-outlet right ventricle	Uhl anomaly

involves keeping the single ventricle as the systemic ventricle and connecting the right atrial blood flow to the pulmonary arteries (Fontan).

Total Anomalous Pulmonary Venous Return Unobstructed

Total anomalous pulmonary venous return (TAPVR) of the unobstructed type is a result of an anomalous pulmonary vein into which all the pulmonary veins drain. The anomalous pulmonary vein then drains into either the superior vena cava (supracardiac type) or into the coronary sinus (intracardiac type). With the supracardiac type the mediastinum is wide, giving the appearance of a snowman. There is always an atrial septal defect, which then causes partially unoxygenated blood to flow systemically.

Tricuspid Atresia

Tricuspid atresia (TA) has been called the great mimic. Characteristically, it is a right-sided ob-

structive lesion due to the atretic tricuspid valve with shunting of the blood across the obligatory atrial septal defect and resultant decreased pulmonary blood flow. However, when there is a ventricular septal defect, there is enough pulmonary blood flow to result in the appearance of an admixture lesion.

Double-outlet Right Ventricle

Double-outlet right ventricle (DORV) has both the aorta and pulmonary artery arising from the right ventricle. There is always a ventricular septal defect, so that blood passes from the left ventricle to the right ventricle and then out the pulmonary artery or the aorta. In addition, systemic venous return blood can also pass from the right ventricle into either the aorta or pulmonary artery, resulting in cyanosis of the patient. The radiographic appearance can be difficult to distinguish from a ventricular septal defect when the thymus obscures the cardiac margins.

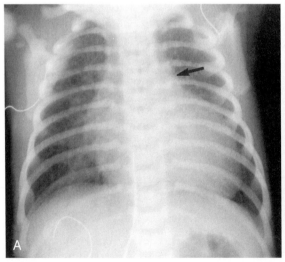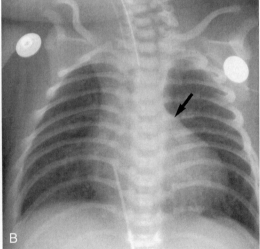

Figure 4–1. A and **B,** Typical findings in two patients with a cyanotic shunt (transposition of the great vessels) showing a concave pulmonary outflow tract *(arrow)* and prominent pulmonary vessels, as well as lack of thymus shadow due to stress.

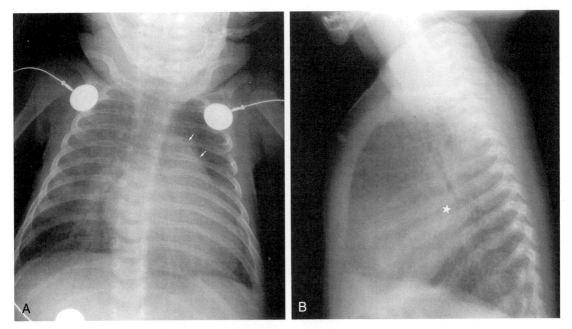

Figure 4–2. A, Frontal view showing an enlarged cardiac silhouette with large pulmonary vessels and prominent pulmonary outflow tract *(arrows).* **B,** Lateral view shows large left atrium *(star)* as is typical of a ventricular septal defect, which is a type of acyanotic shunt.

RADIOGRAPHIC FINDINGS IN RIGHT-SIDED OBSTRUCTIVE LESIONS

Radiographically, the cardiac silhouette is enlarged and the pulmonary vascularity is decreased (Fig. 4–3) so that the lungs look too black (look on the lateral examination behind the heart and in front of the spine to assess for oligemia; it looks too black). The cardiac silhouette may have an uplifted apex, which is due to right ventricular hypertrophy. Unfortunately, normal chest films taken with some lordotic positioning can produce a similar apparent uplifted apex. The classic appearance of the right-sided obstructive lesion can be changed by therapeutic maneuvers, as with prostaglandin therapy, which keeps the ductus arteriosus open. This therapy allows for left-to-right shunting to occur and causes pulmonary vascularity to be present.

Tetralogy of Fallot

Routine tetralogy of Fallot (TOF), which consists of a ventricular septal defect, overriding aorta, right ventricular hypertrophy, and right ventricular infundibular stenosis, usually does not present with cyanosis in the neonatal period. It is usually identified because the neonate has a murmur, which results in the performance of a cardiac echo. The right ventricular outflow tract obstruction is not that severe at first, so the right-to-left shunting does not occur early. However, if the right ventricular outflow tract obstruction is severe, the shunting will occur in the neonatal period and the patient will be cyanotic. There is an association of right aortic arch in approximately 25 percent of these patients.

Critical Pulmonary Valve Stenosis

Critical pulmonary valve stenosis consists of a dysplastic pulmonary valve that results in severe right-sided obstruction. Right-to-left shunting occurs through a patent foramen ovale (PFO) and through the patent ductus arteriosus (PDA) if there are no other intracardiac shunts.

Pulmonary Valve Atresia with Intact Ventricular Septum

Pulmonary valve atresia with an intact ventricular septum (IVS) (Fig. 4–3) is the more extreme version of critical pulmonary valve stenosis. No blood can cross from the right ventricle to the pulmonary arteries. As a result the pulmonary arteries are small and diminutive, and the right ventricle is tiny and hypertrophied. The right atrium is dilated because of tricuspid regurgi-

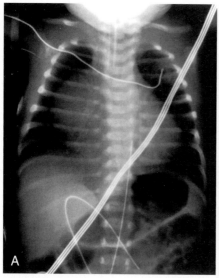
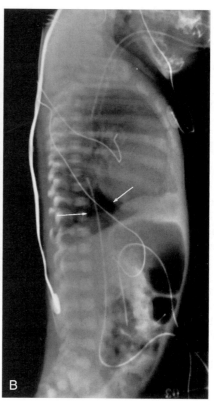

Figure 4–3. A and **B,** Frontal and lateral view of a patient with a severe right-sided obstructive lesion (pulmonary valve atresia with intact ventricular septum) showing a large cardiac silhouette and lungs that are oligemic. To best appreciate the oligemia, the area behind the heart and in front of the spine on the lateral view is the location to observe lack of vascularity *(arrows).*

tation. Right-to-left shunting then occurs as before either through PDA, PFO, or intracardiac shunt.

Tricuspid Atresia

As mentioned previously, the usual presentation of tricuspid atresia is as a severe right-sided obstructive lesion. There is an obligatory shunt at the atrial level. The right ventricle is usually hypoplastic to nonexistent. The right heart border is unusually straight because the right atrium moves over to take up the place normally occupied by the right ventricle.

Ebstein Anomaly

Ebstein anomaly results when there is atrialization of the right ventricle with displacement of the tricuspid valve down into the right ventricular chamber. The tricuspid valve is dysplastic and incompetent, so there is massive tricuspid regurgitation and resultant massive enlargement of the right atrium. When the neonate presents with this lesion, the classic description of the cardiac silhouette on plain radiograph is the "wall-to-wall" heart, because it is so large as a result of the right atrium. In addition, these neonates frequently present with arrhythmias, as well.

Uhl Anomaly

Uhl anomaly is a rare lesion that consists of a dysplastic right ventricular wall that has been compared to a piece of paper in thickness ("parchment" right ventricle). This dysplastic right ventricle acts as a severe right-sided obstructive lesion since it doesn't function. As with other right-sided obstructive lesions, right-to-left shunting occurs through similar pathways.

Chapter 5

The Normal Neonatal Abdomen

ABDOMINAL EXAMINATIONS

After the chest film the abdominal film is the second most frequently ordered examination in the neonate. As in the chest, two views of the abdomen comprise an adequate abdominal examination. These two views include a frontal view and a lateral view with a horizontal beam, such as a cross-table lateral or left-side-down decubitus abdominal view. The horizontal beam film will help to determine the presence or absence of air-fluid levels and the presence or absence of free intraperitoneal air. If the neonate is a newborn, a cross-table lateral view (if the chest is included) is the preferred image, since the vertebral bodies, the sternal-manubrial ossification centers, and the presence or absence of pneumothorax can be better assessed on this view (Fig. 5–1). For subsequent abdominal examinations, the decubitus view is preferred over the cross-table lateral view.

TECHNICAL FACTORS

As in the chest, technical factors must be considered before pathology can be definitively identified. Rotation artifact does not cause as serious a problem as it does in the chest. Rotation can be assessed by looking at the pelvis to determine if it is seen straight on or not. Sometimes rotation is severe enough to make tubes and catheters seem to be in other locations than what was originally thought. For example, an umbilical venous catheter may be projecting to the left because of rotation and, therefore, appear as though it is in the aorta (Fig. 1–2).

The abdomen should be exposed such that the vertebral disc spaces are evident and the lung bases can be seen without the aid of an accessory light or "hot light." If the lungs can be seen well enough on the abdominal film, an assessment of lung inflation should be made. Hyperinflated lungs can cause depression of the hemidiaphragms. This gives an artificial impression of organomegaly by projecting the liver and spleen much more inferiorly than they actually are.

EVALUATING THE NEONATAL ABDOMEN

Tubes and Lines

Tubes and lines need to be assessed. Bladder catheters (if opaque) usually coil over the expected location of the bladder. Umbilical vessel catheters course in the abdomen. As stated before, the umbilical artery catheter (UAC) courses inferiorly before heading in a cephalad direction (Fig. 5–2). Optimal location for the UAC is either in the midthoracic aorta (T6–T9) or below the level of the renal arteries, which are approximately at the level of L1–L2. The umbilical vein catheter (UVC) courses in a cephalad direction from the cord and should lie just above the liver in the inferior aspect of the right atrium. Enteric tubes should be projecting in the stomach if the tube is an orogastric one. The tube should project in a transpyloric location if the tube is for feeding in a transpyloric location. This location usually is across the midline and is posterior in position if a lateral is obtained. Sometimes contrast material needs to be injected into the transpyloric tube to assure its location.

Bony Abnormalities

Bony abnormalities such as vertebral anomalies need to be assessed as with the chest. In particular, the sacral segments should be identified. For example, any sacral anomalies may be associated with anorectal malformations. Tiny punctate calcifications along the spine can be seen in congenital stippled epiphyses or coumadin embryopathy. The shape of the pelvis needs to be assessed since some dwarfs have unusual and classic appearances to the pelvis. In Down syndrome the pelvis may have an unusual "Mickey Mouse ears" appearance. The iliac wings are seen more straight on than usual, and the acetabular roofs are flatter than normal in these cases (Fig. 5–3).

Abdominal organ location and estimations of their size should be completed. When the sides of the abdomen are bulging with displacement of

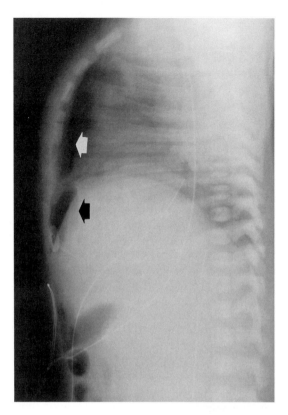

Figure 5–1. Cross-table lateral view of chest and abdomen showing both pneumothorax *(white arrow)* and free intra-peritoneal air *(black arrow)*. Umbilical vessel catheters can be seen as well as sternal ossification centers and vertebral bodies.

Figure 5–2. Frontal and lateral views of patient with infantile respiratory distress syndrome showing the course of umbilical vessel catheters: UAC *(stars)* and UVC *(asterisks)*.

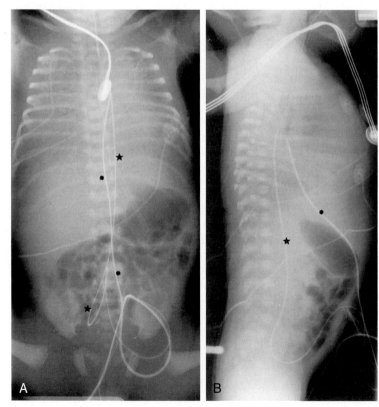

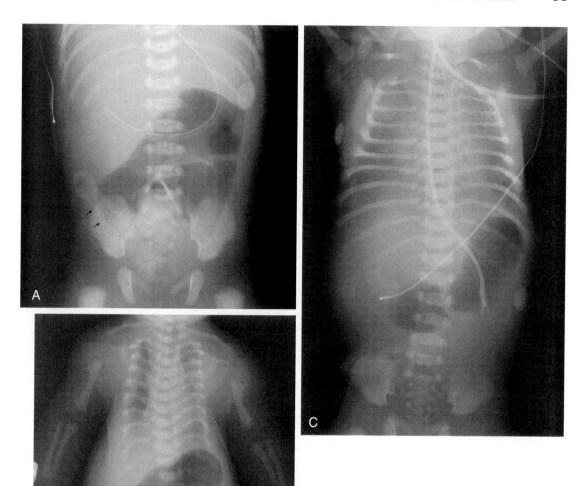

Figure 5–3. A, Neonate with bowel obstruction who has normal appearing bones of the lumbosacral spine and pelvis. Note the umbilical cord clamp *(arrows).* **B,** Patient with asphyxiating thoracic dystrophy with unusual appearance to the pelvis with inferior bony spur seen *(arrow).* **C,** Patient with Down syndrome associated with duodenal atresia, neonatal pneumonia, and the typical "Mickey Mouse ears" pelvis.

the bowel gas inferiorly and somewhat medially, then hepatosplenomegaly should be diagnosed (Fig. 5–4). Also the location of the organs is important. If the liver seems to go all the way across the abdomen and the stomach is midline or on the opposite side from the cardiac apex, consider situs ambiguus (i.e., polysplenia or asplenia).

Calcifications

Calcifications in the abdomen at birth are usually in the liver and result from congenital infection or portal venous thromboemboli (Fig. 5–5). Other calcifications in the abdomen can be seen with meconium peritonitis (Fig. 5–6), which implies that there was an in utero perforation usually

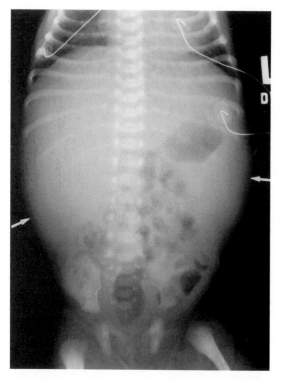

Figure 5–4. Bulging flanks *(arrows)* indicative of hepatosplenomegaly in this patient with congenital infection.

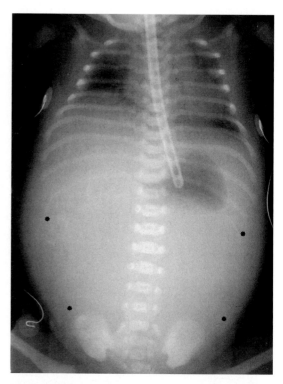

Figure 5–6. Faint calcification *(asterisks)* seen throughout abdomen consistent with meconium peritonitis.

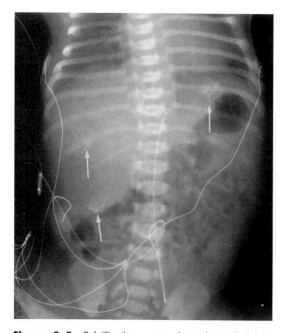

Figure 5–5. Calcifications seen throughout the liver *(arrows)* and confirmed on ultrasound. The exact etiology is unknown but probably represents calcified portal venous thromboemboli.

due to a bowel obstruction that may or may not still be present. Calcification in the position of the colon occurs when there is mixing of meconium and urine in utero, which is seen in anorectal malformations. Usually, it is seen in a male infant.

Properitoneal Fat Stripe

The properitoneal fat stripe is a linear lucency seen along the sides of the abdomen (Fig. 5–7). It is not as lucent as intraluminal bowel gas or free intraperitoneal air. This fat stripe is not seen routinely in premature infants but is present either in infants of diabetic mothers or in large infants. This fat stripe is important when assessing for the presence of ascites. With marked ascites, the bowel is displaced away from the fat stripe.

Abnormal Air Collections

Lucencies over the liver could be from air in vessels, biliary system, or free in the peritoneal cavity. Vasculature air is usually portal venous air that has a branching pattern that extends to the periphery of the liver (Figs. 5–8 and 1–9). Biliary air is seen centrally only. Note: To distinguish

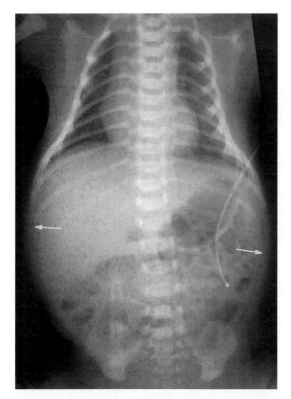

Figure 5–7. Properitoneal fat stripe *(arrows)* in this Down syndrome patient who demonstrates the typical bell-shaped thorax.

portal venous air from biliary air, think of the direction of blood flow (to the periphery of the liver) when compared with the direction of bile flow (to the porta hepatis region). Free intraperitoneal air can be identified on a supine abdominal examination by the observation of different shades of gray over the liver. If there is enough air, the outline of the falciform ligament can be seen (Fig. 5–9) as well: the "football sign."

To confirm the presence or absence of free air, a decubitus view is most helpful because the free air, if present, floats up over the liver laterally (Fig. 5–10A and B). Since there is rarely bowel gas over the liver, it is relatively easy to visualize the free air. On a cross-table lateral view of the abdomen, free air can be seen, but it can be much more difficult to see. Small amounts of air are seen on this view as the telltale triangle of lucency present between loops of air-filled bowel (Fig. 5–10C).

Bowel Gas Pattern

The last part of the neonatal abdomen assessment consists of an evaluation of the bowel gas pattern. In the neonate the small and large bowel cannot be differentiated except by position. The

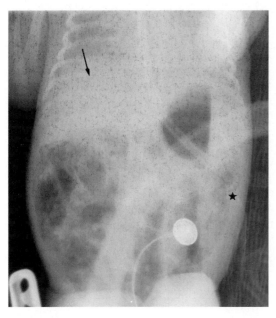

Figure 5–8. Left-side-down decubitus view of abdomen in patient with necrotizing enterocolitis and portal venous air *(arrow)*. Bubbly appearing lucencies of bowel gas *(star)* are pneumatosis intestinalis.

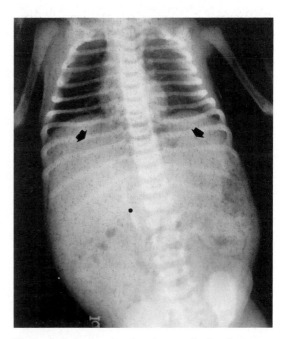

Figure 5–9. Supine view showing two shades of gray over the liver *(arrows)* due to massive pneumoperitoneum. Air is also outlining the falciform ligament as well *(asterisk),* producing the "football sign." The bubbly appearance to the bowel is a result of pneumatosis intestinalis in the patient suffering dead bowel from midgut volvulus.

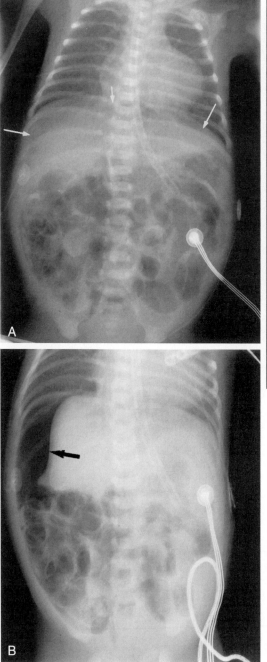

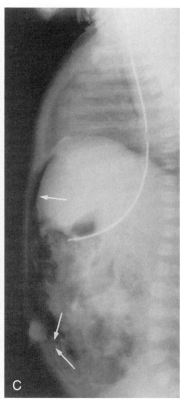

Figure 5–10. Supine, lateral decubitus, and cross-table lateral views showing free intraperitoneal air. **A,** Supine view shows lucency over liver *(arrows)*. **B,** Decubitus view shows air lateral to liver *(arrow)*. **C,** Cross-table lateral view shows air anterior to liver and between loops of bowel *(arrows)*, the "telltale triangle."

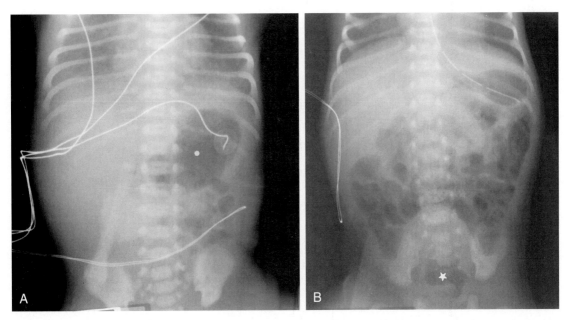

Figure 5–11. A, Gas is seen in the stomach in a normal infant by 30 minutes *(asterisk)* and then on into the rectum **(B)** by 12 hours *(star)* after birth.

gas seen in the left upper quadrant should be stomach. That seen in the pelvis is usually the rectum. The width of the bowel (not stomach) should be no wider than the transverse dimension of the lumbar vertebral bodies. Usually gas is seen in the stomach of a neonate within 30 minutes after birth (Fig. 5–11A) and in the rectum within 12 hours (Fig. 5–11B). A sedated infant who may not be swallowing or one who is extremely ill and has an ileus as a result can affect this pattern. If gas has not reached the anus by 24 hours, then a bowel obstruction must be considered.

Chapter 6

The Neonate with an Abdominal Mass

MOST COMMON MASSES

Abdominal masses in the neonate are usually benign and renal in origin. More and more masses are discovered in the neonate because of prenatal ultrasound. Ultrasound is the postnatal imaging modality of choice followed by abdominal computerized tomography (CT), if necessary. The plain abdominal radiograph is not necessary in the evaluation of the neonatal abdominal mass. All the film shows, as a rule, is the effect of the mass on the normal abdominal soft tissues but gives no clue as to the location of origin of the mass.

RENAL LESIONS

Ureteropelvic Junction Obstruction and Multicystic Dysplastic Kidney

The two most common renal lesions are the ureteropelvic junction obstruction (UPJ) and the multicystic dysplastic kidney (MCDK). Ultrasound can make this differentiation. UPJ shows lucencies in the kidney (which represent the dilated renal pelvis and calyces) that interconnect (Fig. 6–1). MCDK shows lucencies in the kidney that don't interconnect (which represent the dysplastic cysts connected together by abnormal parenchyma) and are called a "bunch of grapes" (Fig. 6–2). MCDK can be associated with UPJ on the other side in approximately 30 percent of cases.

Nuclear medicine is frequently done in both entities, but it is not performed before a few months of age. Before this time the neonate's kidney function is normally decreased compared with an older infant. In UPJ obstruction, a radionuclide renogram demonstrates the obstruction by showing continued accumulation of the radiotracer in the obstructed renal pelvis. The study also gives important information about the remaining function of the obstructed kidney. In MCDK the renogram shows no function on the affected side.

OTHER MASSES

Mesoblastic Nephroma

Mesoblastic nephroma is a mass of the kidney that looks solid on ultrasound, that is, echogenic and indistinguishable from Wilms tumor. Treatment involves nephrectomy where the pathologist makes the differentiation.

Ovarian Cyst

An ovarian cyst can cause an abdominal mass in the neonate because the ovaries are intraabdominal in the neonate. On ultrasound the cyst is a sonolucent mass except when torsion of the ovary is involved. The cyst can then appear as a mass of mixed echogenicity (Fig. 6–3).

Hydrometrocolpos

Hydrometrocolpos is fluid present in an obstructed uterine cavity. On ultrasound, this mass

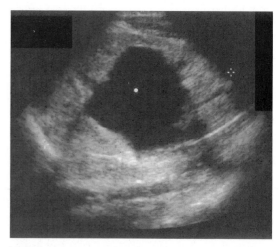

Figure 6–1. Ureteropelvic junction obstruction in a neonate. The kidney is demarcated by the cursors. The central black area represents the dilated renal pelvis (asterisk).

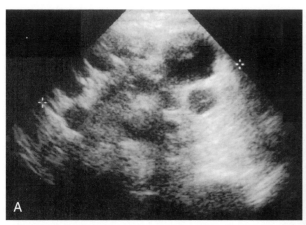

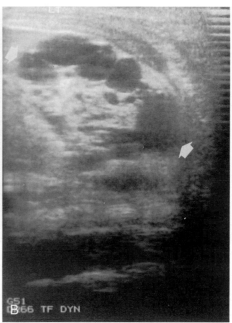

Figure 6–2. Two examples of multicystic dysplastic kidney. The kidney is demarcated by the cursors **(A)** and by arrows **(B).** The black rounded areas represent cysts that don't communicate and are surrounded by dysplastic parenchyma.

is located in the midline and is a sonolucent mass that extends out of the pelvis.

Duplication Cysts and Mesenteric Cysts

Duplication cysts and mesenteric cysts can occur anywhere in the abdomen. Duplication cysts most commonly arise from the ileum. Ultrasound shows a sonolucent collection of fluid.

Neuroblastoma

Neuroblastoma rarely presents in the neonate. However, when it is present, it is usually widespread with metastases to the liver. Ultrasound shows echogenic masses in the liver and wherever the neuroblastoma has metastasized in the abdomen. CT (Fig. 6–4) may be helpful for assessing the extent of tumor spread once it has been investigated by ultrasound.

Figure 6–3. Complicated ovarian cyst with a fluid/fluid level due to hemorrhage *(white arrows).* The irregularity along the inferior wall of the cyst was infarcted ovary *(black arrows).* The cyst extended from the patient's liver to the iliac crest.

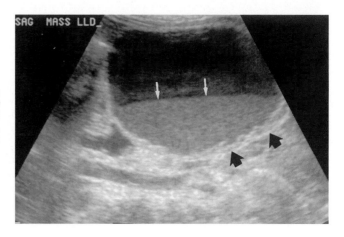

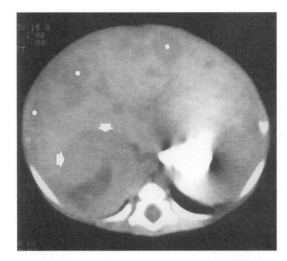

Figure 6–4. Congenital neuroblastoma arising in the right adrenal *(arrows)* with diffuse metastases throughout the liver *(asterisks).*

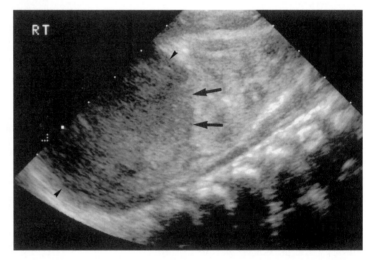

Figure 6–5. Right adrenal hemorrhage *(arrowheads)* causing mass effect on the superior pole of the right kidney *(arrows).* The hemorrhage is homogeneously echogenic at this stage and will ultimately become sonolucent.

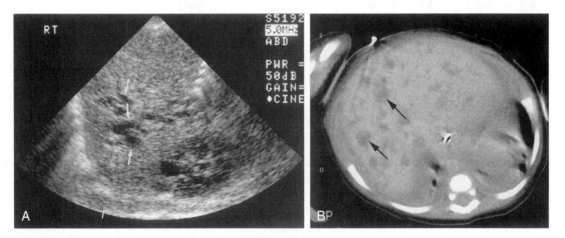

Figure 6–6. Ultrasound **(A)** of the liver in the diffuse form of hemangioendothelioma showing dilated vascular structures in the liver *(arrows).* On precontrast CT **(B)** the hypoattenuating areas *(arrows)* in the liver represent the diffuse form of this entity.

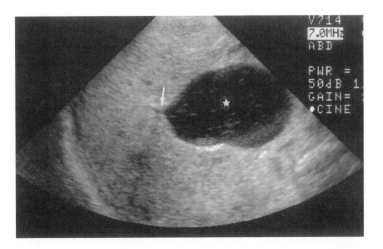

Figure 6–7. Longitudinal view of liver showing black area (choledochal cyst) in the region of the porta hepatis *(asterisk)*. To confirm the origin of the cyst, it has to communicate with the biliary tree *(arrow)* and be separate from the gallbladder.

Adrenal Hemorrhage

Adrenal hemorrhage occurs in the neonate for unknown reasons. Possible etiologies include birth trauma, sepsis, and hypoxia. The hemorrhage is more commonly seen on the right. The classic presentation of an adrenal hemorrhage is that of no symptoms in an infant in whom a renal ultrasound was performed for unrelated reasons. Initially the adrenal hematoma is echogenic and causes a mass effect on the superior pole of the kidney (Fig. 6–5). With time the mass becomes sonolucent and decreases in size. Eventually, the mass calcifies.

Hemangioendothelioma

Hemangioendothelioma causes liver enlargement and is a cause of high output congestive heart failure (see Chapter 3). The lesion can be diffuse or focal in the liver. Therapy consists of treatment for the congestive heart failure. With time the hemangioendothelioma shrinks in size with less shunting of blood through the lesion. On ultrasound (Fig. 6–6A), prominent vascular structures are seen in the liver, and there is frequently evidence of arteriovenous shunting on Doppler ultrasound. CT shows several hypoattenuating structures in the diffuse form (Fig. 6–6B).

Choledochal Cyst

Choledochal cyst can be a cause of obstructive jaundice in the neonate. There are traditionally four types of choledochal cyst, with the fifth type being Caroli disease. Fusiform dilatation of the common bile duct, Type 1, is the most common. The other types are discussed in Chapter 9. Ultrasound shows a sonolucent mass in the region of the porta hepatis that is separate from the gallbladder (Fig. 6–7). The cyst communicates with the intrahepatic biliary tree and frequently causes intrahepatic biliary dilatation. Nuclear medicine biliary imaging scan confirms the connection of the cyst with the biliary tree and shows subsequent excretion of the radiopharmaceutical into the gut.

Cyst Associated with Biliary Atresia

Cyst associated with biliary atresia can be mistaken for a choledochal cyst, but the cyst does not communicate with the intrahepatic biliary tree. There may or may not be a gallbladder visualized. Ultrasound shows a sonolucent mass in the region of the porta hepatis that does not communicate with the intrahepatic biliary tree. Nuclear medicine biliary imaging scan shows no excretion of the radiopharmaceutical into the cyst or gut.

Chapter 7

The Neonate with Abdominal Distension

There are two main reasons for abdominal distension in the neonate: bowel obstruction from a mechanical reason and ileus, which is a functional obstruction. With both causes of distension, the infant can vomit bile or there can be increased residual volumes of food in the stomach. Diagnosis of mechanical bowel obstruction in the neonate rests on the nonvisualization of gas in the expected location of the rectum after the first 24 hours. If incomplete mechanical obstruction is present, such as with duodenal stenosis, there is a discrepancy in the size of the bowel, with the more proximal bowel (proximal to the stenosis) being dilated out of proportion to the more distal bowel. It is this discrepancy in size of bowel loops, as well as the absence of gas distally, that makes the diagnosis of a mechanical obstruction (Fig. 7–1). The diagnosis of ileus is made when there is uniform dilatation of all bowel loops including loops all the way to the rectum (Fig. 7–2).

MECHANICAL BOWEL OBSTRUCTION

Gut Atresias

Gut atresias can be encountered in any portion of the bowel, from the esophagus to the colon. Of the small bowel atresias, jejunal and ileal atresias are the most frequently encountered. Duodenal atresia is about half as common and is associated with Down syndrome. Colon atresia is uncommon. Esophageal atresia occurs slightly less than jejunoileal atresias.

Tracheoesophageal fistula (TEF) with or without esophageal atresia (EA) or esophageal atresia

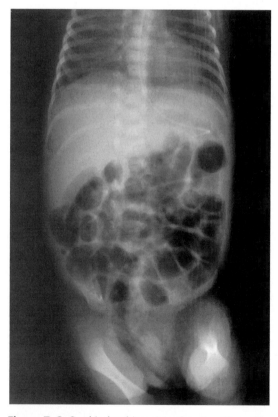

Figure 7–2. On this decubitus view, there is uniform dilatation of all bowel loops with gas seen all the way to the rectum, indicating an ileus.

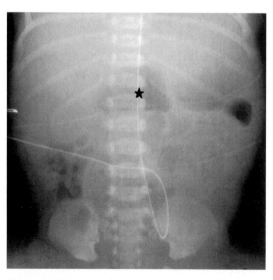

Figure 7–1. Duodenal stenosis demonstrated by the dilated proximal duodenum *(star)* and nondilated more distal bowel in this patient with Down syndrome. Note the "Mickey Mouse ears" pelvis as a clue to the underlying syndrome.

with or without tracheoesophageal fistula presents in the neonatal period when the orogastric tube cannot be inserted in those patients that have esophageal atresia. Those that have tracheoesophageal fistula have abdominal distension as well, due to air-distended loops of bowel. Five different combinations of this disorder are possible. The most common of this disorder is with a proximal EA and distal TEF (Fig. 7–3). The next most common type is that of isolated EA and no TEF. Other less common types are isolated TEF without EA, EA with proximal TEF only and no distal connection, and EA with both a proximal and distal TEF.

The initial evaluation of the entity is made with plain radiographs. When the most common type is present, the proximal esophageal pouch is localized either by air in it or by the orogastric tube that is stuck in the pouch. Air in the stomach proves that there is a distal TEF. With isolated EA, there is no gas in the stomach (Fig. 7–4). With isolated TEF, the orogastric tube goes down to the stomach, but there is gaseous distension of bowel with an air esophagram and, frequently, right upper lobe aspiration. Isolated TEF is usually diagnosed with barium in the esophagus. This last entity is uncommon.

When EA or TEF is present, the VACTERL association must also be considered. VACTERL is an acronym for an association of abnormalities involving different parts of the body: V = vertebral anomaly, A = anorectal malformation, C = congenital heart lesion, TE = tracheoesophageal fistula, R = renal anomaly or rib anomaly, L = limb abnormality. When one of the "letters" is present, a thorough search for the remainder must be considered.

The etiology of the small bowel atresias, with the exception of duodenal atresia, is thought to be a vascular accident with resultant infarction and subsequent atresia of the involved bowel. Duodenal atresia is thought to be due to a failure of recanalization of the bowel lumen. Duodenal atresia may be associated with annular pancreas, which is a ring of pancreatic tissue surrounding the duodenum. This latter diagnosis is usually only discovered at surgery, although occasionally it can be seen on ultrasound.

With gut atresias, distended loops of bowel filled with air are seen on plain abdominal radio-

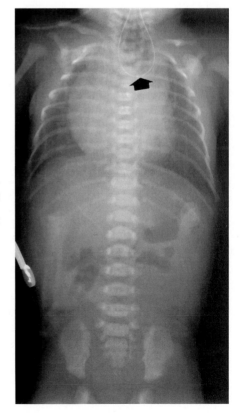

Figure 7–3. Proximal esophageal atresia pouch is demonstrated by the looped orogastric tube *(arrow)*. There is a distal tracheoesophageal atresia present as evidenced by air in the stomach and proximal gut. This patient also has congenital heart disease and unusual ribs as part of the VACTERL association.

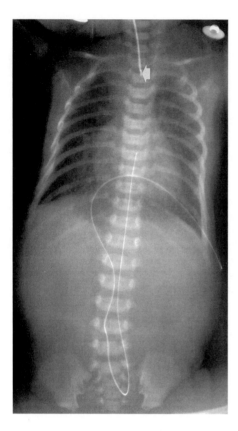

Figure 7–4. Down syndrome patient (note bell-shaped chest) with proximal esophageal atresia as demonstrated with orogastric tube *(arrow)* and no distal tracheoesophageal fistula, which results in a gasless abdomen.

graphs. The more proximal the obstruction, the fewer the loops that will be seen (Fig. 7–5). For example, duodenal atresia shows two air-filled structures: stomach and duodenal bulb. On horizontal beam films there are two air-fluid levels: the "double bubble." If more than two loops are seen, then the obstruction is more distal. As long as the number of loops is countable, no other imaging studies are needed. If loops are too numerous to count, then the obstruction is more distal. When a hugely dilated loop is seen, the diagnosis of atresia is almost certain, with the atresia distal to the huge loop (Fig. 7–6). An enema may need to be done to distinguish a distal gut atresia from other entities that will be discussed later. A contrast enema in a patient with ileal atresia shows an empty colon that is unusually small, a "microcolon," with reflux of contrast into an empty terminal ileum up to the atresia (Fig. 7–7). If the atresia is in the jejunum, the caliber of the colon will be relatively normal because of the passage of intestinal secretions from the more distal bowel into the colon. If the plain film shows a jejunal atresia but the enema shows a microcolon, there are other more distal atresias present as well (Fig. 7–8).

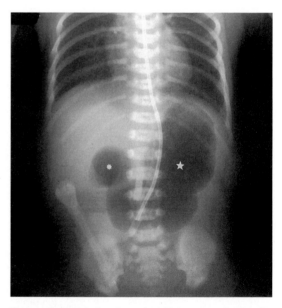

Figure 7–5. Duodenal atresia with gas seen in the distended stomach *(star)* and duodenal bulb *(asterisk)* but not seen distally.

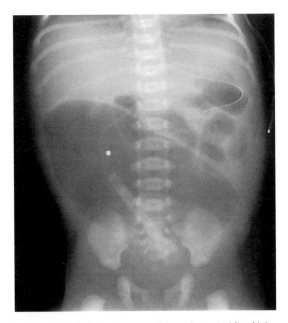

Figure 7–6. Patient with a small bowel atresia (distal jejunal) showing a hugely dilated loop of bowel *(asterisk)*, which was proximal to the atresia.

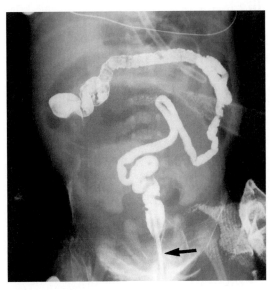

Figure 7–7. Contrast enema showing a microcolon, that is, small colon that is not much larger than the caliber of the enema tube *(arrow)*.

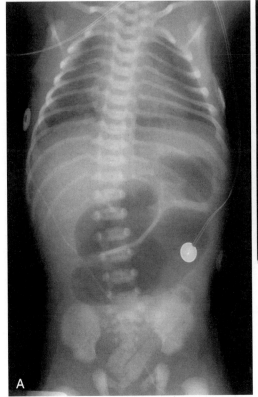

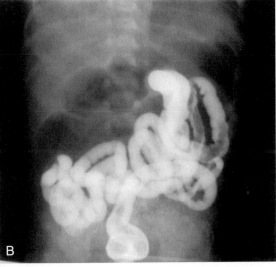

Figure 7–8. A, Plain radiograph showing only a few dilated loops of bowel indicative of a jejunal atresia. **B,** However, contrast enema shows a microcolon that indicated that more distal atresia is present.

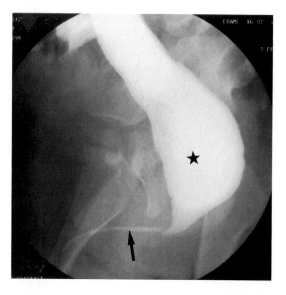

Figure 7–9. Contrast study in a male with high imperforate anus demonstrating the fistula from the colon *(star)* to the urethra *(arrow).*

Imperforate Anus

Imperforate anus is related to abnormal separation of the genitourinary system and the hindgut. The imperforate anus malformation is divided into high and low lesions depending on whether the colon terminates above or below the pelvic sling. Those low lesions usually have some sort of perineal fistula on physical examination. The high lesions have no visible perineal abnormality and have an internal fistula to the urinary tract in males (Fig. 7–9) and to the genital tract in females. The low lesions are treated with perineal surgery and the high lesions are treated with a colostomy.

Radiology helps to identify the level of the colon if it is not clear on physical examination. With ultrasound, the meconium-filled colon can be visualized. If the end of the colon is measured as 1.5 cm or less from the perineum, then the lesion is a low malformation. Radiology can help in the evaluation of other associated abnormalities consistent with the VACTERL association. Renal anomalies, sacral anomalies, and spinal cord abnormalities are the most frequently associated problems. In the neonate, both the kidney and spinal cord evaluations can be performed with ultrasound. The sacral vertebral body evaluation is performed with the aid of plain radiographs.

Meconium Plug Syndrome

Meconium plug syndrome is seen in sedated term infants and is a problem with colon inertia.

Clinically, the infants have distended abdomens and fail to pass meconium after 24 hours. Usually the infant starts to vomit, as well. Hirschsprung disease is associated with meconium plug in 30 percent of cases. The presence of Hirschsprung disease is confirmed pathologically when there are no ganglion cells in the distal colon. Therefore suction rectal biopsy to look for ganglion cells is usually recommended for these patients.

Plain radiographs show dilated gut throughout the abdomen. The procedure of choice to diagnose meconium plug syndrome is to perform a contrast enema, usually with hypertonic contrast material. The contrast helps not only to diagnose this condition but also to treat the infant by relieving the obstruction. (Note: To use this contrast material, the infant should be well hydrated and should have a patent intravenous line in place before the examination begins.) The hypertonic contrast draws water into the lumen of the colon, which lubricates the meconium and helps the infant pass the plug. The colon is relatively normal in caliber and displays a long-filling defect (Fig. 7–10), which is the meconium plug. Usually at the end of the procedure the infant passes the plug on the fluoroscopy table.

Neonatal Small Left Colon Syndrome

Neonatal small left colon syndrome is also a colon inertia problem. It is highly associated with infants of diabetic mothers. As the name implies, the appearance of the colon is that of a microcolon in the region of the descending, sigmoid, and

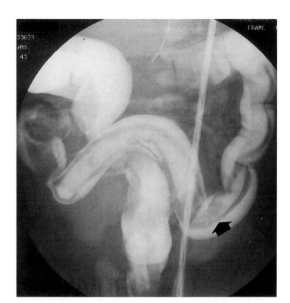

Figure 7–10. Meconium plug syndrome seen with a contrast colon exam showing a relatively normal caliber colon with a large filling defect (meconium plug) within it *(arrow)*.

rectal colon. The left colon is small because it is unused. At the splenic flexure, the colon suddenly dilates, which gives the impression of a transition zone as seen with Hirschsprung disease. For this reason, some people think that this entity is a variant of meconium plug syndrome and, therefore, has a risk of Hirschsprung disease. Whether suction rectal biopsy is indicated in these patients is controversial. Once the diagnosis has been made by contrast enema, the patient usually starts to stool in a few days.

Meconium Ileus

Meconium ileus is an entity seen in 10 to 15 percent of patients with cystic fibrosis (CF). The patient has CF until proven otherwise when this diagnosis is made. On plain radiograph, there are dilated loops of bowel too numerous to count, sometimes a bubbly appearance to the meconium, usually a lack of air/fluid levels because the meconium is too viscous to make air/fluid levels, and a disorganized appearance to the bowel loops (Fig. 7–11). Ultrasound of the abnormal meconium

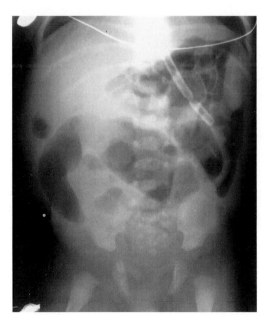

Figure 7–11. Left-side-down decubitus view showing an unusual bowel gas pattern in a patient with meconium ileus. There are several loops present, some dilated, spread over the abdomen. No air-fluid levels are present on the decubitus image.

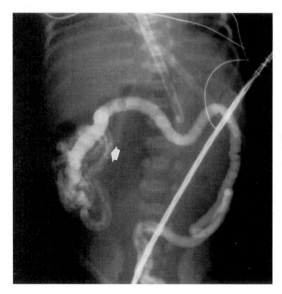

Figure 7–12. Contrast enema showing an empty microcolon but meconium pellets filling the terminal ileum *(arrow)*, which is where the obstruction is in typical meconium ileus.

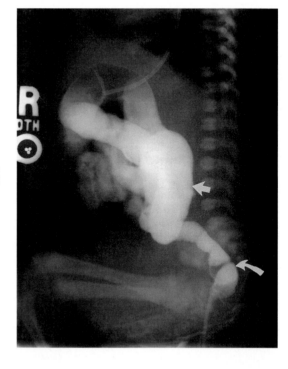

Figure 7–13. Lateral view of patient with Hirschsprung disease showing small caliber of distal colon *(curved arrow)* compared with more proximal colon *(arrow)*.

can show echogenic bowel contents and can help in the preenema evaluation of the patient. Contrast enema performed with hypertonic water-soluble contrast shows a microcolon with several filling defects (pellets of abnormal meconium) in the terminal ileum (Fig. 7–12). If the contrast is refluxed retrograde far enough, the small bowel is dilated proximal to the filling defects. The purpose of the enema is to diagnose and also to treat the obstruction by helping to flush out the abnormal meconium pellets. It is sometimes difficult to distinguish meconium ileus from ileal atresia. In general, if ileal atresia is present, air/fluid levels will be present on the plain abdominal radiograph. Ultrasound will not demonstrate the highly echogenic meconium as seen with meconium ileus. Contrast enema will show a microcolon, but the terminal ileum will be extremely small and empty without the filling defects as seen in meconium ileus.

Hirschsprung Disease

Hirschsprung disease is one in which there is a lack of ganglion cells, usually in the distal 10 centimeters, although any length of bowel could be lacking ganglion cells. The lack of these cells causes the involved segment of colon to be in constant spasm and remain small, in turn causing obstruction to the more proximal colon, which dilates outward as it peristalses against the obstruction. Because of the obstruction the patient may present with enterocolitis and resultant pneumatosis, which is a serious and potentially fatal complication. On contrast enema, usually done with barium and with the patient in the lateral position, the discrepancy in caliber size (i.e., transition zone between the small, spastic, aganglionic segment and the more proximal dilated segment) can be appreciated (Fig. 7–13). However, sometimes it is difficult to see this transition zone in a neonate. Rectal biopsy is done for definitive diagnosis. Since the transition zone is not always in the distal colon, the caliber discrepancy can be anywhere in the colon. When the whole colon is aganglionic, the colon can be a microcolon with the terminal ileum dilated and filled with meconium.

In summary, there are three causes of the appearance of a microcolon on contrast enema: meconium ileus, ileal atresia, total colon aganglionosis.

ILEUS

Ileus can be simulated by uniform distention resulting from iatrogenic bagging for ventilation or from continuous positive airway pressure (CPAP). The presence of ileus is nonspecific (Fig. 7–14) and can be due to sepsis, electrolyte imbalance, gastroenteritis, milk allergy, and necrotizing enterocolitis, among others. Ileus is the first radiographic manifestation of necrotizing enterocolitis (NEC), but since its presence is so nonspecific, it is of little use in the initial diagnosis of NEC.

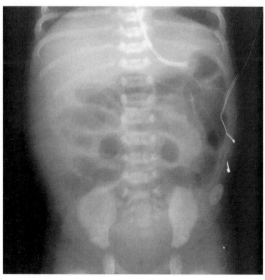

Figure 7–14. Supine view showing ileus as demonstrated by distended loops of nearly the same caliber. Frequently no gas is seen in the rectum with necrotizing enterocolitis, giving the false impression of mechanical obstruction.

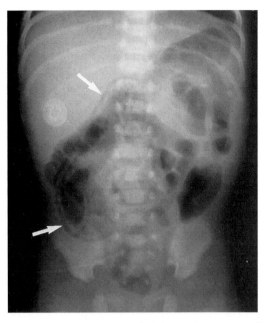

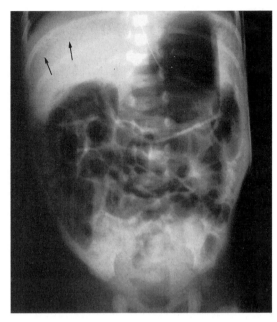

Figure 7–15. Supine view of abdomen in patient with necrotizing enterocolitis. Bubbly appearing lucencies of bowel gas are pneumatosis intestinalis *(arrows).*

Figure 7–16. Decubitus view in patient with necrotizing enterocolitis and portal venous gas in the liver causing faint, ill-defined lucencies over the liver *(arrows).*

Necrotizing Enterocolitis

Pneumatosis intestinalis is the hallmark of NEC. Pneumatosis is air in the bowel wall that can be either bubbly or linear in appearance (Fig. 7–15). A bubbly pattern in the bowel contents is usually only seen during the first 24 hours of life and after 14 days. If bubbles are seen in this time interval, especially if there is an ileus, then NEC should be considered. Sometimes a prone film will help to dilate the ascending and descending colon because these areas are posterior in location. Once the colon is dilated, the diagnosis of pneumatosis is made more easily.

Air in the portal vein (Fig. 7–16) is also con-firmatory evidence of pneumatosis, since the pneumatosis can escape the bowel wall and enter the superior mesenteric vein (SMV). The SMV and the splenic vein join to make up the portal vein. Once the diagnosis of NEC is made, serial films need to be obtained, usually at 6-hour intervals, to evaluate for surgical intervention, that is, for free intraperitoneal air, fixed dilated loop, which means dead loop, or portal venous air, a relative indication for surgery. Usually the films taken are a supine abdomen and left-side-down decubitus abdominal view. Filming ceases when the pneumatosis has resolved or the patient has gone to surgery.

Chapter 8

The Neonate or Young Infant with Vomiting

BILIOUS VOMITING

All babies spit up or vomit at times. When there is associated apnea, wheezing, desaturation, or weight loss, an imaging investigation should be obtained to exclude anatomic causes of this condition. Clinically, the color of the vomitus is important. For example, bilious (greenish yellow) vomiting is an ominous sign, but it is not specific. Patients that have an ileus can have bilious vomiting due to backing up of intestinal contents with resultant bilious emesis. Patients with bowel obstruction can have bilious emesis, as well. If there is no obvious reason on plain radiograph for the patient to have bilious vomiting, the baby needs an imaging evaluation immediately. The definitive examination should be a barium upper gastrointestinal (UGI) examination to exclude midgut volvulus.

Midgut Volvulus

Bilious vomiting in a previously well neonate results from midgut volvulus until proven otherwise. Midgut volvulus is a neonatal disease in the vast majority of cases. Eighty to eighty-five percent of cases occur in the neonatal period, and one third of these occur in the first week of life. Patients with midgut volvulus have malrotation of the midgut. Those patients with only malrotation will show that the duodenal-jejunal junction is in an abnormal location on UGI examination (Fig. 8–1). The normal location is just to the left of the spine at approximately the L1 pedicle level (Fig. 8–2). With volvulus causing complete obstruction, the UGI film shows a beaklike appearance to the duodenum (Fig. 8–3). If the patient is not completely obstructed, the barium will proceed distal to the beak, and the barium column will appear to circle around inferiorly. Frequently, midgut malrotation is associated with Ladd's bands, which are peritoneal bands that the body has formed anomalously to try to fixate the bowel. There is often obstruction with these bands in a similar location to midgut volvulus.

In patients undergoing abdominal ultrasound for indications other than bilious vomiting, midgut malrotation can be suggested on the basis of the ultrasound by seeing the superior mesenteric vein lie to the patient's left of the superior mesenteric artery in the transverse plane. Normally, the vein lies to the patient's right of the artery. However, absence of this feature does not entirely exclude midgut malrotation and its presence is not definitive of midgut malrotation, but an UGI film should be obtained to exclude its presence.

Other Duodenal Pathology

There are other much less common causes of obstruction that lead to bilious vomiting in the infant such as duodenal web and duodenal stenosis. On barium studies a duodenal web has the appearance of a vertical, linear filling defect in the duodenum at the junction of the second and third portions of the duodenum. The web can have a pinpoint opening in it, which causes the obstruction (Fig. 8–4A). Duodenal stenosis is, as the name implies, a narrowing in the duodenum at the junction of the first and second duodenum. On plain film studies the duodenum proximal to

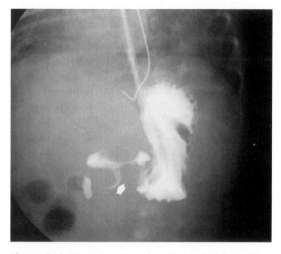

Figure 8–1. Neonate with malrotation and midgut volvulus as demonstrated by the abnormal location of the duodenal-jejunal junction *(arrow)*. The circling appearance of the bowel is characteristic of volvulus that is not completely obstructed.

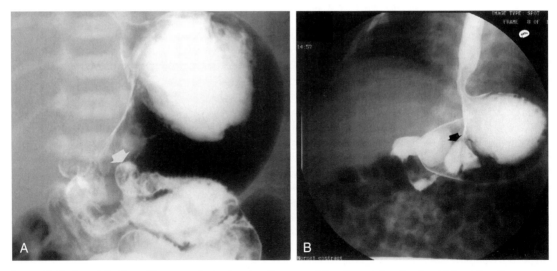

Figure 8–2. A and **B,** Two different patients showing the normal location of the duodenal-jejunal junction on UGI examination *(arrows).*

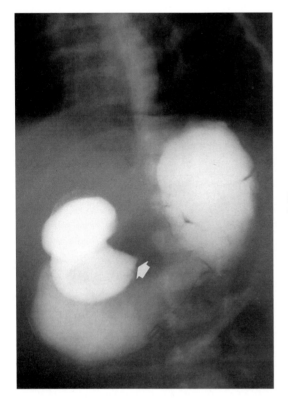

Figure 8–3. Midgut volvulus with total obstruction demonstrating a beaklike appearance to the barium course *(arrow).*

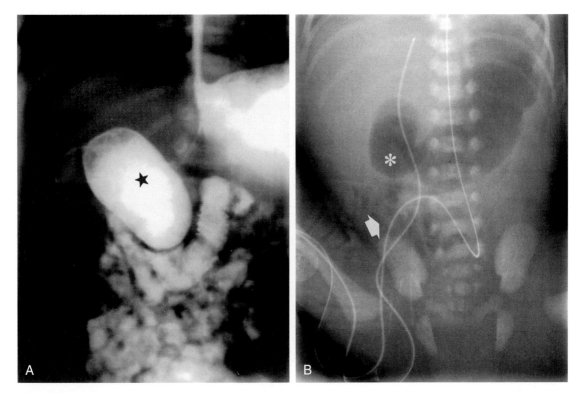

Figure 8–4. A, UGI examination in patient with duodenal web that has a small opening in it with resultant enlargement of the proximal duodenum *(star)*. **B,** Duodenal stenosis with dilated duodenum *(asterisk)* seen with decompressed gut seen more distally *(arrow)*.

the stenosis is dilated with the distal duodenum decompressed (Fig. 8–4B). Sometimes these duodenal entities are incidentally seen on ultrasound when the patient is being evaluated for pyloric stenosis. The dilated, fluid-filled proximal duodenum is the first clue to duodenal pathology. When this pathology is suspected, a barium study is then undertaken for definitive diagnosis.

NONBILIOUS VOMITING

Gastroesophageal Reflux

The most common cause of nonbilious vomiting in the neonate is gastroesophageal reflux. All babies reflux to a certain degree because of the obtuse angle that the esophagus makes with the stomach (Fig. 8–5). As the infant ages, the angle becomes more acute, and usually the episodes of reflux diminish. Evaluation of gastroesophageal reflux should be reserved for those patients who have associated symptoms.

Plain chest radiograph of the infant can suggest massive reflux by the presence of an air esophagram (Fig. 8–6). Included in the differential diagnosis of an air esophagram are air swallowing,

burp in progress, and, infrequently, the presence of an isolated tracheoesophageal fistula ("H-type" TEF without esophageal atresia).

Functional imaging is most commonly done with the UGI examination. Besides reflux, the UGI film can show swallowing abnormalities (Fig. 8–7) and any anatomic abnormality that might predispose the patient to reflux. Observation of reflux is performed for 5 minutes with the patient content and the stomach full.

Another imaging modality for reflux evaluation is the nuclear medicine gastric emptying and reflux study. This study evaluates the patient for an hour and is more physiologic than a barium study, since real food that has been radiolabeled is given to the patient. Both an assessment of the presence of gastroesophageal reflux and an estimation of gastric emptying time can be made. Some investigators believe that a prolonged gastric emptying time (normal is at least half of the radiolabel emptying in an hour) puts the patient at risk for delayed reflux. The problem is that the study is three to four times more expensive than the barium exam and the resolution of the images is not sufficient to evaluate anatomical abnormalities (Fig. 8–8) or swallowing incoordination.

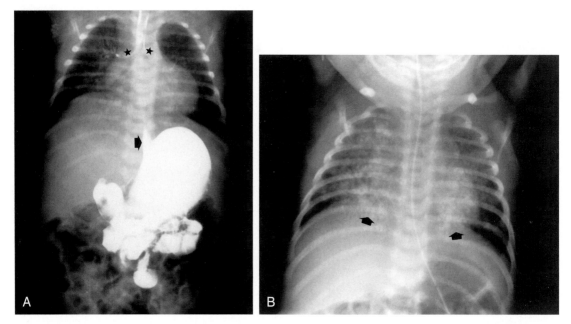

Figure 8–5. A, Neonate with gastroesophageal reflux *(arrow)* and subsequent tracheal aspiration *(stars)*. **B,** Chest radiograph taken after the UGI examination. The white areas in the lungs are sites of barium aspiration to the lungs *(arrows)*.

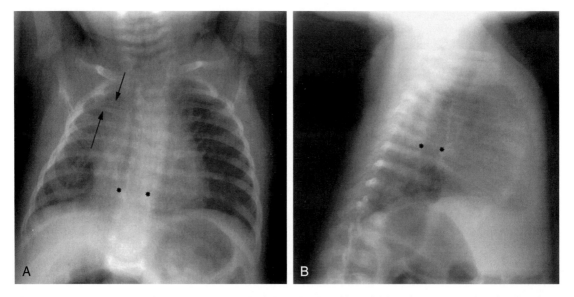

Figure 8–6. Air esophagram *(between asterisks)* on both frontal **(A)** and lateral **(B)** in this patient with isolated tracheo-esophageal fistula. Patient also has rib anomalies on right *(arrows)*. (Note: VACTERL association.)

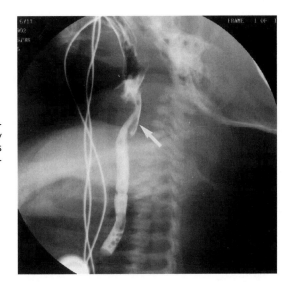

Figure 8–7. Lateral view of swallowing. The diverticulum-like area in the proximal esophagus *(arrow)* was caused by a perforation in the posterior wall of the hypopharynx. This finding resulted in swallowing incoordination and subsequent aspiration.

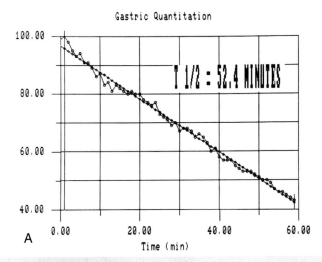

Figure 8–8. A, Gastric emptying time calculated with the aid of the computer showing a normal emptying where more than half the gastric contents emptied by 1 hour. **B,** Images over the stomach *(arrow)* showing no evidence of reflux.

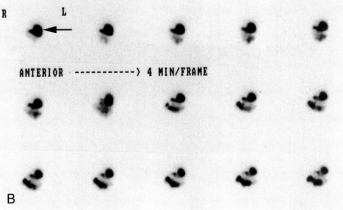

Aspiration of the gastric contents is rarely seen with this procedure, because the aspiration has to be of a large enough quantity and stay in the lungs long enough for the imaging camera to resolve it.

Hypertrophic Pyloric Stenosis

Another cause for nonbilious vomiting in the young infant is hypertrophic pyloric stenosis (HPS). This entity is typically seen in males around 4 to 8 weeks of age but can be seen as early as 1 week and as late as several months after birth. The diagnosis can be made clinically by palpating the hypertrophied muscle, which has the feel of an olive. However, this palpation is difficult even with experienced hands. Imaging is frequently required to diagnose this condition.

Although not necessary, a plain abdominal radiograph (KUB) is sometimes obtained for evaluation of HPS (Fig. 8–9). Characteristic findings on the KUB are gastric distention out of proportion to the rest of the abdominal bowel gas pattern, which is nonspecific because frequently babies swallow air and can reproduce this appearance. The second finding is the "caterpillar sign," which is a distended stomach showing peristaltic waves of the stomach that is trying to peristalse against the pylorus.

Ultrasound is the mainstay of imaging in many institutions. It is relatively quick, requires no NPO status, and evaluates the whole muscle. On ultrasound, the muscle wall is the most sensitive measurement in making the diagnosis of HPS (Fig. 8–10). It is relatively hypoechoic when compared with the lumen of the pyloric channel. The diagnostic measurement is 4 millimeters, although anything over 2 millimeters is abnormal, but HPS may not be present. The whole muscle diameter is the next most sensitive measurement at 13 millimeters, but anything over 11 millimeters is abnormal. When the muscle is seen in a transverse plane, it has the appearance of a target with the hypoechoic muscle wall surrounding the relatively hyperechoic mucosa and mucous in the lumen. The length of the muscle is the least sensitive measurement at 17 millimeters. When the muscle hypertrophies, it elongates and curves, making measurement difficult. Sonographically, another feature of HPS is that the pylorus does not open and close, as does a normal pylorus. (Note: An easy way to remember the measurements diagnostic of HPS: 4 + 13 = 17.)

A barium UGI examination is a method still employed for the diagnosis of HPS. However, it does involve radiation and puts the patient at increased risk of aspiration. Most of the time, the patient is so obstructed that it takes a long time to diagnose the hypertrophied muscle. This causes an increased radiation dose to the patient.

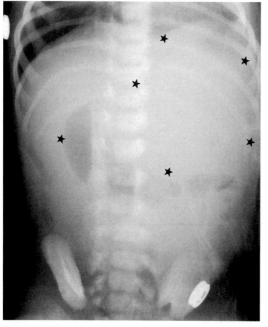

Figure 8–9. Left-side-down decubitus image showing the approximate location *(stars)* of a dilated, mainly fluid-filled, stomach and little gas seen distally indicative of gastric outlet obstruction: hypertrophic pyloric stenosis.

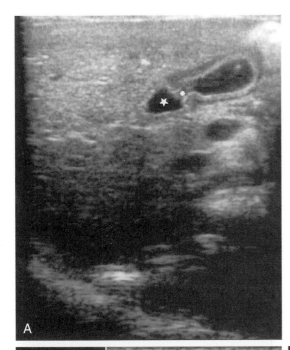

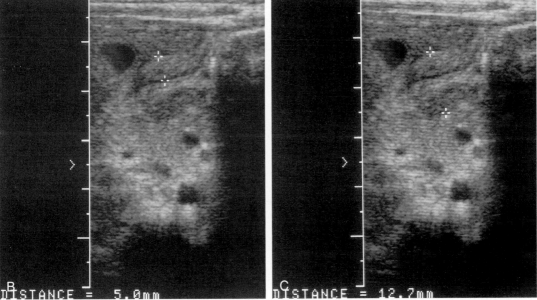

Figure 8–10. A, Normal pylorus at ultrasound *(asterisk)* that is fluid-filled and open. The black triangular collection is duodenal bulb *(star)*. **B,** Abnormal pylorus with the hypertrophied muscle wall demarcated by cursors. **C,** The whole transverse muscle demarcated by cursors.

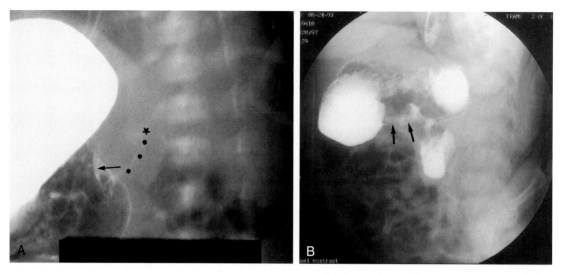

Figure 8–11. A, UGI film showing hypertrophic pyloric stenosis with mass effect seen on antrum *(arrow)*, string sign of narrowed and elongated pylorus *(asterisks)*, and faint visualization of duodenal bulb *(star).* **B,** Another patient with pyloric stenosis on UGI film demonstrating elongated pylorus *(arrows).*

To do the study safely, an orogastric tube must be passed into the stomach to instill the barium and to aspirate it back out if the diagnosis is made.

The diagnosis on UGI examination includes visualizing the following signs:

- The antral beak sign, which is seen as barium heads into the hypertrophied muscle
- The antral shoulder sign, which is caused by a mass effect of hypertrophied muscle on the antrum

- The string sign, which is caused by barium passing through the elongated channel of the hypertrophied muscle

The mass effect on the duodenal bulb, which is caused by the hypertrophied muscle mass impressing upon the bulb, must also be seen (Fig. 8–11). Sometimes the hypertrophied muscle can be appreciated *en face* even before the string sign is demonstrated if compression is used on the antrum of the stomach.

Chapter 9

The Neonate with Jaundice

Jaundice is a common condition in the neonate. Most of the time, the jaundice is self-resolving. However, when the jaundice persists, imaging must be employed to exclude a surgically correctable lesion such as biliary atresia or a choledochal cyst. Included in the differential diagnosis of these lesions are neonatal hepatitis and cholestasis problems associated with intravenous hyperalimentation.

OBSTRUCTIVE JAUNDICE

Biliary Atresia

Biliary atresia is loss of patency of the biliary tree that progresses over time from an extrahepatic location to an intrahepatic one. Etiology is unknown but may be related to some viral insult. Imaging evaluation is usually with ultrasonography (US) first to exclude a cause of extrahepatic obstruction other than biliary atresia, such as a choledochal cyst. The diagnosis of biliary atresia can be inferred by US, which frequently shows a small, contracted, or absent gallbladder (although 20 percent can have a normal gallbladder) and no evidence of biliary obstruction. In a fasting patient, a gallbladder measuring less than 1.5 centimeters is highly suspicious for biliary atresia.

Definitive imaging is then performed with nuclear scintigraphy using technetium-99m iminodiacetic acid (IDA) agents, frequently DISIDA. The exam usually is performed after the patient has been given phenobarbital b.i.d. at a dose of 5 mg/kg/d for 3 to 7 days before the injection. The images in biliary atresia show good hepatic uptake of the radiopharmaceutical but no excretion out of the biliary tree and no gut excretion 24 hours later (Fig. 9–1).

Surgery is performed in this entity where an attempt is made to establish biliary flow, usually by the creation of some sort of portoenterostomy. Ultimately the patient usually requires hepatic transplantation.

Choledochal Cysts

Choledochal cysts are the result of cystic dilatation of the extrahepatic bile duct. The etiology of these cysts is thought to arise from the anomalous insertion of the common bile duct into the pancreatic duct with subsequent reflux of pancreatic enzymes up the duct. The lesion is a premalignant one of which there are five types. Type 1A is localized dilatation of the common bile duct below the cystic duct. Type 1B is dilatation of the common bile duct and intrahepatic ducts. Type 2 is an eccentric diverticulum of the common bile duct. Type 3 is focal dilatation of the common bile duct as it passes through the wall of the duodenum (choledochocele). Type 4 is multiple, dilated, nonobstructive, intrahepatic and extrahepatic bile ducts. When the intrahepatic ducts are involved, the condition is also known as Caroli disease (type 5).

The classic triad of abdominal pain, jaundice, and palpable right-sided mass is usually not seen in the neonate and young infant. Many of the cases are now diagnosed on prenatal ultrasound. Postnatal ultrasound is the diagnostic imaging modality of choice. Ultrasound easily shows the cystic dilatation of the common bile duct that must be differentiated from the gallbladder (Fig. 9–2A). In addition, US can clearly show the communication of the cyst with the remainder of the intrahepatic biliary tree. In older children, the cyst can be associated with stone formation. Although not usually necessary, confirmatory imaging with radionuclide scintigraphy (technetium-99m IDA) can show the radiotracer in the liver, which then accumulates in the cyst followed by bowel excretion. Intraoperative cholangiography is usually performed to confirm the anatomy of the common bile duct as it enters the pancreatic duct (Fig. 9–2B).

There are two other much more rare conditions that can cause neonatal obstructive jaundice. Biliary hypoplasia, which is also known as Alagille syndrome, can simulate biliary atresia but has a better prognosis. The second is inspissated bile syndrome, which is caused by precipitated bile within the bile ducts (Fig. 9–3). Inspissated bile syndrome is associated with prolonged hyperalimentation and cystic fibrosis. The precipitated bile causes biliary obstruction and is frequently a self-resolving entity once oral feeds are estab-

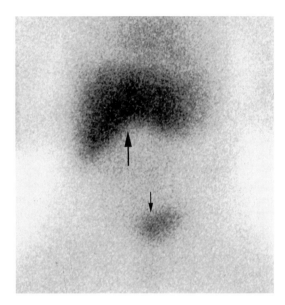

Figure 9–1. Imaging of biliary atresia showing good hepatic uptake *(long arrow)* and persistent urinary excretion in the bladder *(short arrow)* but no bowel excretion.

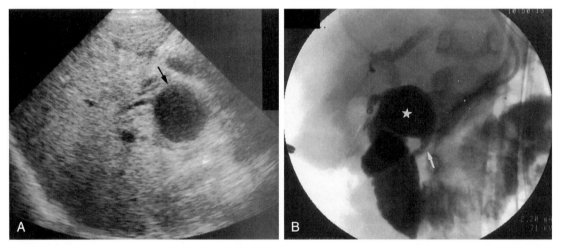

Figure 9–2. A, Choledochal cyst *(arrow)* first seen on prenatal ultrasound and confirmed postnatally. **B,** Intraoperative cholangiogram showing contrast in the cyst *(star)* that then enters the pancreatic duct *(arrow).*

Figure 9–3. Inspissated bile syndrome is seen here as an echogenic focus *(thin arrows)* in a dilated intrahepatic duct. Portal vein is below the duct *(wide arrow).*

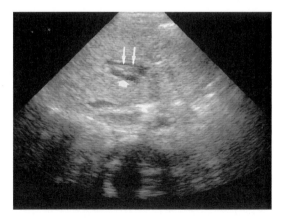

lished. Infrequently, surgical cleansing of the biliary tree may be necessary.

NONOBSTRUCTIVE JAUNDICE

Neonatal Hepatitis

Neonatal hepatitis is to be differentiated from biliary atresia, since this condition is treated medically. A variety of infectious agents have been implicated in this disorder, such as congenital infections and unknown infections. Imaging is usually with ultrasound first to confirm the presence of a gallbladder, which is usually visible in this entity, and to exclude an obstructed cause of jaundice. However, differentiating hepatitis from biliary atresia cannot be done on the basis of the ultrasound.

Definitive imaging is then performed in the same fashion as with biliary atresia. The images in neonatal hepatitis usually show poor hepatic uptake of the tracer with residual blood pool activity present for a prolonged period of time. Gut activity is seen usually within 24 hours as opposed to biliary atresia (Fig. 9–4). In practice, there can be overlap between the findings of biliary atresia and neonatal hepatitis. If biliary atresia has gone unrecognized for long enough with resultant cirrhosis, the nuclear medicine image may mimic the findings of neonatal hepatitis. Conversely, if the hepatic function in a patient with neonatal hepatitis is poor enough, not enough tracer will

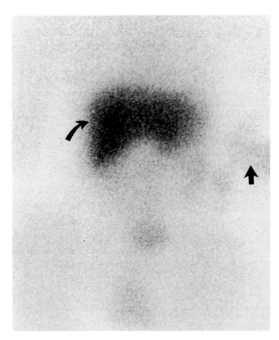

Figure 9–4. Neonatal hepatitis on biliary imaging shows gut excretion, here in an ostomy bag *(arrow)*, by 18 hours. Usually the hepatic uptake *(curved arrow)* is poorer than seen here.

ever get excreted into the gut, and the image may simulate biliary atresia. If either diagnosis is in doubt, liver biopsy can frequently distinguish these two entities.

Chapter 10

The Neonate with an Abdominal Wall Defect

The two main diagnoses in this category are gastroschisis and omphalocele. In general, gastroschisis is a good diagnosis to make; omphalocele is an ominous diagnosis. Gastroschisis is associated with other abnormalities approximately 5 percent of the time. Omphalocele is associated with other anomalies roughly 45 to 75 percent of the time.

GASTROSCHISIS

The diagnosis of gastroschisis is frequently made by prenatal ultrasound, which shows the defect to be to the right of midline and separate from the insertion of the umbilical cord. Loops of small bowel are seen floating in amniotic fluid without a covering membrane. Occasionally, bowel atresias can be associated. The diagnosis is obvious at birth (Fig. 10–1), and imaging plays no part in the diagnosis unless there is an associated atresia present. In those few cases, the air-filled bowel proximal to the atresia will be dilated.

Postoperatively, the bowel gas pattern is disorganized for weeks because gut motility is abnormal for a long time and the gut is malrotated as part of the anomaly. Adhesions can occur once the defect has been closed, but volvulus is rarely seen as a complication. Sometimes even pneumatosis is seen, which is of unknown significance but does not necessarily mean enterocolitis. These patients are usually maintained on hyperalimentation for prolonged periods through a surgically placed central venous catheter.

OMPHALOCELE

The diagnosis of omphalocele is also usually made by prenatal ultrasound, which shows the defect to be midline with the umbilical cord in-

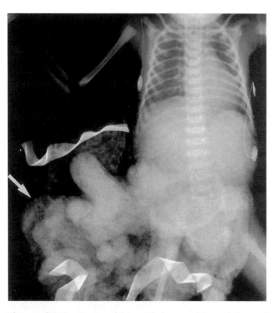

Figure 10–1. Gastroschisis with loops of bowel *(arrow)* seen outside the abdomen.

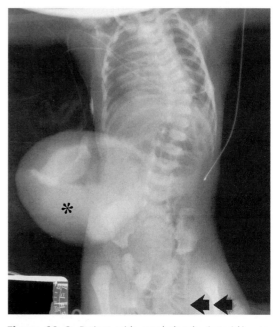

Figure 10–2. Patient with omphalocele *(asterisk)*, narrowed chest, and scoliosis due to abnormal positional forces in utero. Incidental note is made of left-sided inguinal hernia *(arrows)*.

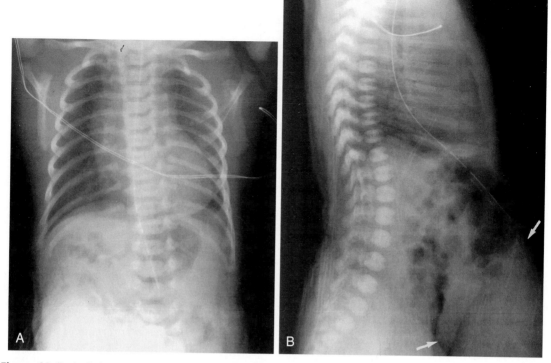

Figure 10–3. A, Patient with a giant omphalocele and a narrow chest appearance. **B,** Lateral view of same patient showing membrane-covered omphalocele *(arrows)*.

serting at the apex of the herniated contents. A membrane surrounds the contents (Fig. 10–2), and usually the liver is contained in omphalocele. Radiographs can aid in diagnosing associated anomalies such as trisomy 18 or possible cardiac anomalies.

In those neonates that have the "giant omphalocele," the thorax configuration is unusual in that the chest is somewhat narrowed and elongated (Fig. 10–3). This thoracic appearance does not necessarily change once the defect has been returned to the abdomen.

Chapter 11

The Neonate with Anuria or Oliguria

Most infants void within 24 hours of birth. Initial evaluation of anuria should occur around 12 hours of birth. Usually this evaluation begins with bladder catheterization. If urine is obtained, no further evaluation is needed. If no urine returns out of the catheter, imaging with ultrasound is the next step. There is no place for intravenous urogram (pyelogram, IVP) in evaluating renal pathology in the neonate. Renal function in these infants is normally about one fourth that of the older child and adult. Visualization sufficient for diagnosis usually is not possible under these conditions.

IMAGING

The normal appearance of kidneys on ultrasound in the premature and term neonate is different from that of adults. The cortex, in at least half of term neonates, is the same echogenicity (isoechoic) as is the liver and spleen. This is because of the increased number of glomeruli in the renal cortex of the term neonate when compared with older infants. Older infants, children, and adults have cortical echogenicities less than adjacent liver and spleen. In addition, the medullary pyramids in the neonate are more prominent and larger (Fig. 11–1). These findings gradually disappear so that the kidneys assume the adult pattern between 6 and 12 months. There is also no visible sinus fat in the neonatal kidney, but its presence doesn't become the adult pattern until adolescence. Premature infants have renal cortices that are hyperechoic compared to the adjacent liver and spleen. The hyperechogenicity is increased the more premature the infant.

The adrenal gland is prominent in the neonate and is approximately one third the size of the kidney. Its appearance is that of an echogenic inner layer over a sonolucent outer layer. The shape is similar to an arrowhead or a V or Y configuration (Fig. 11–2A). When the kidney is absent or ectopic, the adrenal has an elongated appearance (Fig. 11–2B). When the elongated appearance is encountered and the contralateral kidney is normal in size, the ipsilateral kidney is usually ectopic. If the contralateral kidney is hypertrophied, the other kidney is usually absent.

PATHOLOGIC CONDITIONS CAUSING ANURIA AND OLIGURIA

Causes of anuria and oliguria in the neonate include the following: hypoperfusion states, dehydration states, absence of kidneys, urinary tract obstruction, renal vascular thrombosis, dysplastic kidneys, autosomal recessive kidney disease, and precipitation of protein (Tamm-Horsfall protein) in the medullary pyramids.

Acute Tubular Necrosis and Renal Vein Thrombosis

The kidneys typically have a normal appearance in renal arterial thrombosis, mild hypoperfusion states, and dehydration instances. Typically, the cortex is increased in echogenicity in severe hypoperfusion states, as in severe acute tubular necrosis (ATN). Because the normal kidney in the term and preterm neonate is hyperechoic to isoechoic, the diagnosis of ATN by ultrasound can be difficult in these patients. Once the ATN resolves, the kidney returns to normal echogenicity. The normal-sized kidney with loss of the normal cortical-medullary demarcation is most often seen with renal dysplasia. The enlarged kidneys with this loss of demarcation are typically seen in renal vein thrombosis (RVT), where hemorrhage is frequently encountered (Fig. 11–3), and in autosomal recessive polycystic kidney disease.

Obstruction

With obstruction there is separation of the normal renal sinus echoes, resulting in echolucency in this region (Fig. 11–4). If no dilated ureter is

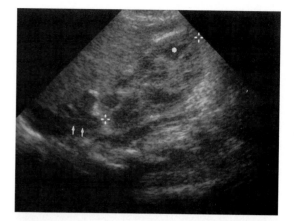

Figure 11–1. Normal longitudinal ultrasound of neonatal kidney as demarcated by the measuring cursors. The black areas in the kidney *(asterisk)* represent renal pyramids. Cephalad to the kidney is the normal adrenal *(arrows).*

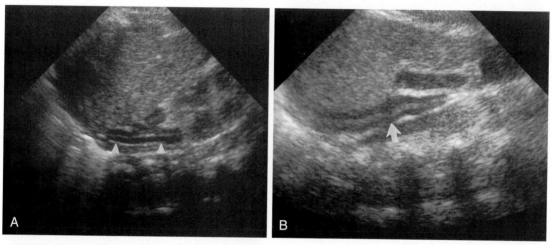

Figure 11–2. A, Normal adrenal with a Y-shape configuration *(arrowheads).* **B,** Elongated adrenal when the kidney is absent or ectopic *(arrow).*

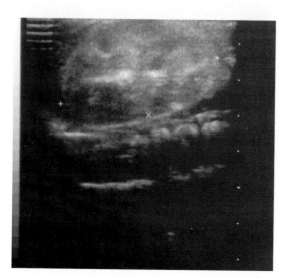

Figure 11–3. A case of renal vein thrombosis in which there is a loss of the normal cortical-medullary demarcation. The bright echogenic foci in the kidney represent areas of hemorrhage. The kidney is demarcated by cursors.

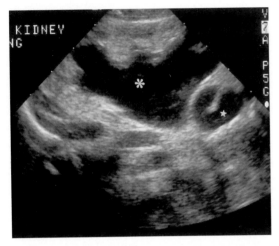

Figure 11–4. Longitudinal view of kidney showing echolucency *(asterisk)*, which is urine, in the renal sinus echoes as well as dilation of the ureter *(star)* in this patient with ureterovesical junction obstruction.

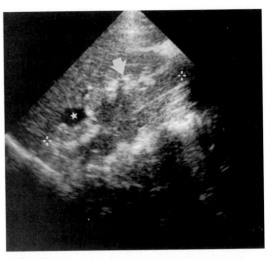

Figure 11–5. Duplication anomaly with two sets of renal sinus echoes, the lower pole *(arrow)* is normal and the upper pole shows dilatation *(star)* secondary to obstruction.

seen, the separation may be the result of ureteropelvic junction obstruction. Physiologic distention of the sinus can occur if the bladder is full, so postvoid images are desired, although not always easy to obtain in the neonate. Vesicoureteral reflux can cause this appearance, as well. If there is an appearance of two sinus echo complexes, then a duplication anomaly of the kidney is suggested (Fig. 11–5). In the classic case of complete duplication, the upper pole obstructs because of ectopic ureteric insertion, and the lower pole refluxes.

Protein Deposition

Precipitation of protein, Tamm-Horsfall protein, in the medullary pyramids is a cause of transient renal dysfunction in the neonate. Sonographically, the pyramids show increased echogenicity (Fig. 11–6) within them that disappears once renal function returns. The differential diagnosis of the echogenic pyramids in the neonate includes infection. In the older infant, the most common cause for this appearance is nephrocalcinosis due to furosemide therapy.

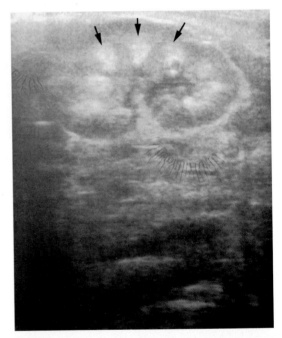

Figure 11–6. Echogenic renal pyramids *(arrows)* due to protein deposition in this neonate.

Chapter 12

The Neonate with Urinary Tract Infection

A urinary tract infection (UTI) in the neonatal period is usually due to some abnormality of the urinary tract. The evaluation of a patient with UTI is renal and bladder sonography followed by voiding cystourethrography (VCUG). The normal renal ultrasound appearance, as is also discussed in Chapter 6, shows an echogenic cortex with prominent echolucent pyramids. The prominent pyramids should not be mistaken for cysts or hydronephrosis.

ULTRASOUND IMAGING

In any child with a UTI, renal sonography is performed during the acute infection to make sure that there is not an obstructed, infected kidney that needs to be drained. Usually, renal ultrasound is normal even when vesicoureteral reflux is present. When abnormality is present, such as separation of the calyceal collecting system echoes (pelvocaliectasis or hydronephrosis), there are three possible explanations: physiologic distention, obstruction, and reflux (Fig. 12–1). Scarring may also be seen as a result of reflux nephropathy. The scarring frequently involves the poles of the kidneys first.

Bladder ultrasound should always be included when renal ultrasound is performed. The normal bladder should be imaged in both transverse and longitudinal planes (Fig. 12–2), and the bladder wall should be measured in the longitudinal dimension. If the bladder is distended, the wall should be no more than 3 millimeters in thickness. If the bladder is not distended, the wall should be no more than 5 millimeters in thickness. Sometimes dilated ureters are seen behind the bladder (Fig. 12–3). Masses in the bladder should be observed for, such as ureteroceles, which are usually associated with duplicated collecting systems but may be draining single collecting systems. The ureteroceles drain and result in obstruction of the upper pole, and there is usually reflux into the lower pole (Fig. 12–4). In the case of ambiguous genitalia, imaging for a uterus behind the distended bladder can be performed. Imaging of the distal colon through a distended bladder in patients with imperforate anus can be obtained, as well.

VOIDING CYSTOURETHROGRAPHY

A VCUG is the next imaging procedure. It is performed after the acute infection has resolved and the patient is no longer symptomatic. This

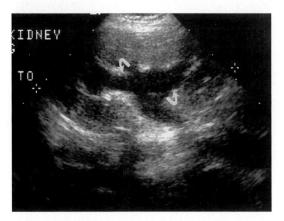

Figure 12–1. Separation of the calyceal collecting system echoes *(arrows)* because of vesicoureteral reflux.

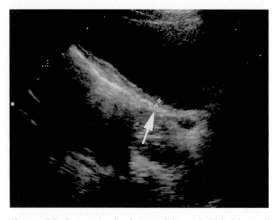

Figure 12–2. Longitudinal view of distended bladder wall being measured *(arrow)* in this plane.

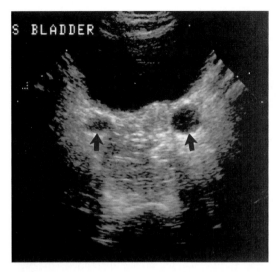

Figure 12–3. Transverse view through bladder showing bilateral dilated ureters *(arrows)* in this infant with bilateral vesicoureteral reflux.

procedure is usually performed 2 to 6 weeks after the acute event to allow residual inflammation to resolve. The normal VCUG should show a distended bladder that is smooth and sharp in outline. Cyclic voiding is performed in infants under 1 year of age. This technique is accomplished by having the patient void around the catheter and then refilling the bladder. Reflux is sometimes brought out only by this technique for reasons not completely understood. Voiding images without the catheter should be obtained in the steep oblique projection in males and in frontal or lat-

eral projection in females (Fig. 12–5). Frequently there is vaginal reflux in females, which is normal but must be separated from the urethral images. Images over the kidneys must be taken post void to evaluate for vesicoureteral reflux. It is important to have the bladder at maximal distention, because reflux sometimes only occurs at maximal distention. Voiding images are equally as important for the same reason. Bladder capacity can be estimated up to age 14 by the formula:

$$(\text{Age in years} + 2) \times 30 = \text{Capacity in milliliters}$$

Vesicoureteral reflux is graded according to the level that the refluxing column of contrast reaches. If the contrast only reaches the ureter, then grade 1 reflux is present. Grade 2 reflux occurs when the contrast reaches the calyceal system, but there is no blunting of the calyces. If the calyces are blunted with slight ureteral dilatation, then grade 3 reflux is present (Fig. 12–6). With ureteral dilatation and tortuosity present, grade 4 reflux has occurred. When there is massive dilatation of both calyces and ureters, then grade 5 is present. Spontaneous resolution can occur in cases of reflux, but the chance of this occurring drops dramatically with the higher grades.

If the screening renal ultrasound shows bilateral hydronephrosis in a male infant, bladder outlet obstruction should be the diagnosis—usually posterior urethral valves (PUV). These infants usually are not diagnosed because of UTI but rather because there was an in utero examination or a noticeable decrease in the urinary stream on voiding. Although much more rare, anterior

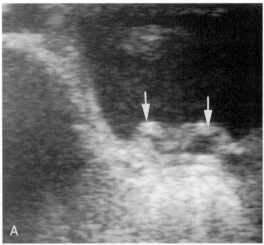

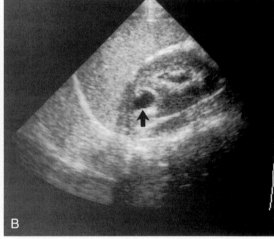

Figure 12–4. A, Transverse view through bladder showing ureteroceles *(arrows)* due to bilateral duplicated systems. **B,** Longitudinal view of one kidney showing the duplicated collecting system echo complex. The ureterocele is draining the upper pole system *(arrow).*

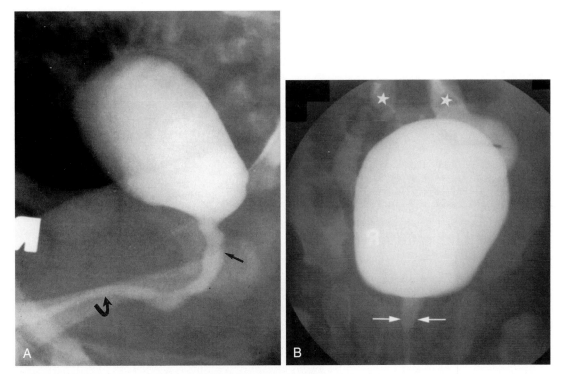

Figure 12–5. A, Normal male urethra in the oblique projection. Posterior urethra is identified by the presence of the verumontanum *(straight arrow)*. Anterior urethra is shown by curved arrow. **B,** Normal female urethra *(arrows)* is equivalent to the posterior urethra in males. Note the bilateral vesicoureteral reflux *(stars)*.

urethral valves cause the same obstruction to the bladder with subsequent bilateral hydronephrosis. Other diagnoses such as neurogenic bladder and dysfunctional voiding are potential causes, but these usually cause problems in the older infant and child. In a female infant, bilateral hy-

dronephrosis is usually due to vesicoureteral reflux.

The renal ultrasound not only can show the dilated collecting systems but also dilated ureters and the thick-walled bladder that are present in patients with bladder outlet obstruction. If PUVs

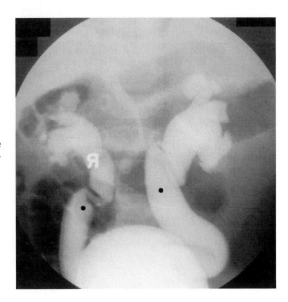

Figure 12–6. Bilateral massive vesicoureteral reflux (grade 5) with dilated, redundant ureters *(dots)* and marked calyceal dilation.

are present, sometimes the ultrasound can visualize the dilated posterior urethra as well (Fig. 12–7). VCUG is then performed to observe the valves and to see whether or not reflux is present, since it occurs in 50 percent of these cases. In the other 50 percent, the hydronephrosis is caused by obstruction at the ureterovesical junction as a result of such a thick-walled bladder. The thick wall is shown on VCUG by marked wall irregularity (Fig. 12–8). The voiding portion of the examination is critical for diagnosis. With valves (Fig. 12–9), the posterior urethra is markedly dilated and the anterior urethra is not. (Note: The obstruction is only to antegrade flow and not in a retrograde direction, so patients with PUVs can be catheterized without difficulty.) Anterior urethral valves show an obstruction in the anterior urethra (Fig. 12–10).

When prenatal ultrasound has shown hydronephrosis, either unilateral or bilateral, a follow-up postnatal examination needs to be done. Exact timing of the postnatal examination is uncertain. Historically, the examinations were performed 3 days after birth to allow the relatively dehydrated state of the newborn to resolve. For severe renal abnormalities this waiting period may not be necessary. If this examination is abnormal, then a follow-up ultrasound and VCUG need to be performed. Controversy exists over the follow-up of normal postnatal examinations.

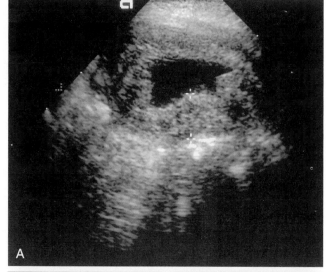

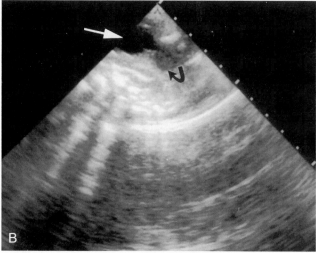

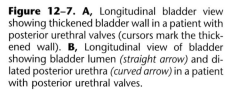

Figure 12–7. A, Longitudinal bladder view showing thickened bladder wall in a patient with posterior urethral valves (cursors mark the thickened wall). **B,** Longitudinal view of bladder showing bladder lumen *(straight arrow)* and dilated posterior urethra *(curved arrow)* in a patient with posterior urethral valves.

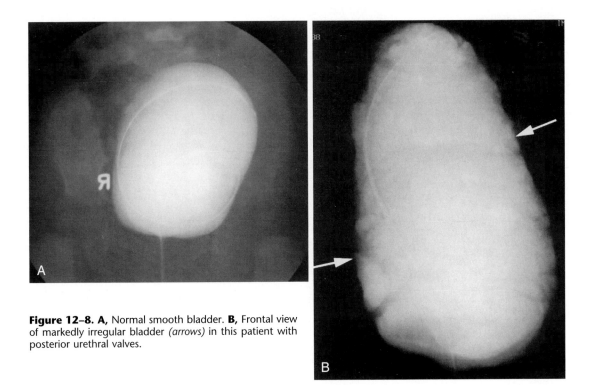

Figure 12–8. A, Normal smooth bladder. **B,** Frontal view of markedly irregular bladder *(arrows)* in this patient with posterior urethral valves.

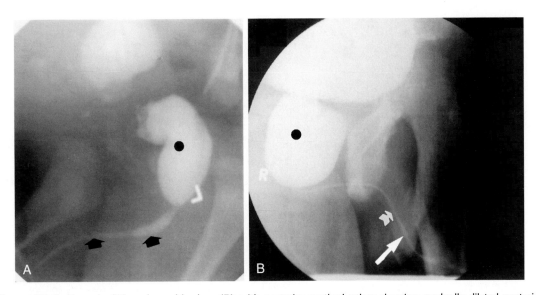

Figure 12–9. Neonate **(A)** and an older boy **(B)** with posterior urethral valves showing markedly dilated posterior urethra *(dots)* and small anterior urethra *(arrows)*.

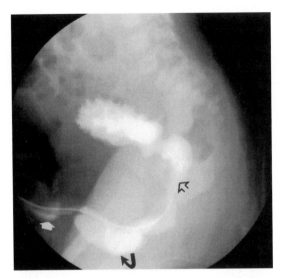

Figure 12–10. Anterior urethral valve *(curved arrow)* with posterior urethra demonstrated *(open arrow)* and remainder of anterior urethra *(closed arrow)* seen.

RENOGRAM

If the VCUG is normal but the screening ultrasound had shown calyceal separation, the next procedure of choice is a nuclear medicine renal function study (i.e., a renogram). The procedure is usually performed later, around 3 months of age. This procedure involves the intravenous injection of a radiopharmaceutical with imaging over the kidneys obtained afterward. Furosemide is frequently given to enhance excretion by the kidneys. The computer generates uptake and excretion curves from these images. If no excretion of the tracer occurs, the kidney is obstructed (Fig. 12–11). If there is a slight delay in excretion of the tracer, then the renal collecting system is dilated but not obstructed, which can be termed physiologic distention.

INTRAVENOUS PYELOGRAM

There is no place for an intravenous pyelogram (IVP) in the evaluation of a patient with a UTI unless a ureteral abnormality is suspected. However, this study cannot be performed in the neonatal period because the glomerular filtration rate of a neonate is so much lower than in older infants and adults. The excretion of contrast is therefore suboptimal for visualization on plain radiographs. If an IVP needs to be done, waiting several months is ideal for performing an adequate study.

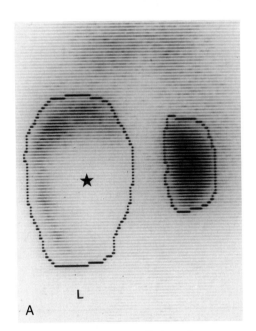

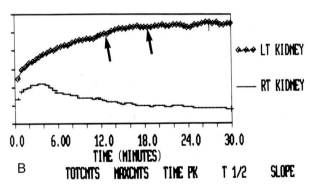

Figure 12–11. A, Images of kidneys from renogram of older infant showing a rim of activity around a "cold" area *(star)* where no activity has been excreted because of obstruction. **B,** Computer-generated curves of both kidneys where tracer accumulates and is never excreted *(arrows)*.

Chapter 13

The Neonate with Anomalies Associated with Underlying Renal Abnormalities

There are many syndromes and anomalies in which renal involvement plays a part. A few of them will be mentioned here.

VACTERL ASSOCIATION

Whenever there is a vertebral anomaly present (Fig. 13–1), a renal ultrasound needs to be performed, because there is a 40 percent incidence of renal abnormality associated. Likewise, in those patients with anorectal abnormality, there is a 50 to 70 percent association of renal abnormalities (Fig. 13–2) in those patients with high imperforate anus and a 15 percent incidence in those with low lesions. In those patients undergoing cardiac evaluation for congenital heart disease, renal imaging should also be done because of the potential for associated abnormalities.

NEUROGENIC BLADDER ASSOCIATION

Patients with myelomeningocele or sacral agenesis (Fig. 13–3) and resultant neuro-

genic bladder usually have a normal renal ultrasound at birth. Later on, the kidneys begin to show abnormality, such as hydronephrosis and decreased size. The decreased size is a result of the neurogenic bladder either because of associated reflux that frequently occurs or because of the obstruction that the neurogenic bladder generates when the wall is highly trabeculated. (Remember: Use latex precautions in these patients.)

TWO-VESSEL CORD ASSOCIATION

Twenty-one percent of the time in neonates, a two-vessel umbilical cord is associated with other abnormalities. Hydronephrosis and dysplastic kidney comprise some of these abnormalities. Without other abnormalities present, evaluation

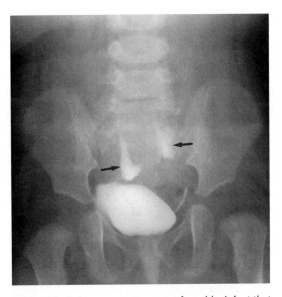

Figure 13–2. Intravenous urogram of an older infant that shows pelvic fused kidneys in this patient with previous isolated esophageal atresia and imperforate anus. The white areas above the bladder are the malrotated collecting systems *(arrows)* filled with contrast.

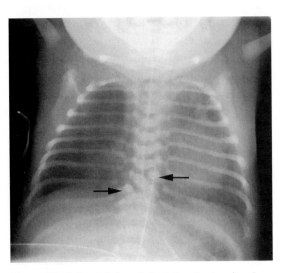

Figure 13–1. Frontal view of chest showing two hemivertebrae *(arrows)*.

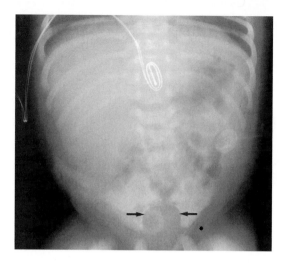

Figure 13–3. Near complete absence of the sacrum with resultant small bony pelvis *(arrows)*. Incidental note is made of dislocated left hip *(asterisk)*.

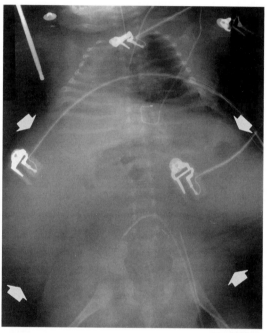

Figure 13–4. Prune belly syndrome with marked bulging of the lateral abdominal walls *(arrows)* due to absence of the abdominal musculature.

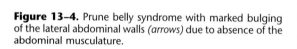

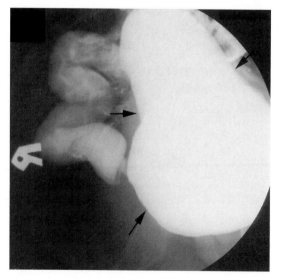

Figure 13–5. Same patient as Figure 13–4 with prune belly syndrome. VCUG shows large bladder *(arrows)* and marked right-sided vesicoureteral reflux.

with renal ultrasound of all patients who have a two-vessel cord is not cost-effective.

PRUNE BELLY SYNDROME

Prune belly syndrome is usually found only in males and consists of the absence of abdominal musculature (Fig. 13–4). These patients have abnormal urinary tracts that consist of a dilated urinary tract including large ureters, bladder, urethra, and bilateral cryptorchidism. Renal sonography shows bilateral hydroureteronephrosis and a distended bladder. Voiding cystourethrography (VCUG) shows vesicoureteral reflux (Fig. 13–5), a dilated and somewhat unusual appearance to the bladder, and a dilated, but nonobstructed, urethra.

BLADDER EXSTROPHY

Exstrophy of the bladder is present when the bladder is open on the anterior abdominal wall. The kidneys are usually normal. The ureteral orifices can be seen as well as the length of the urethra. The radiograph of the pelvis shows an unusual orientation of the iliac bone such that

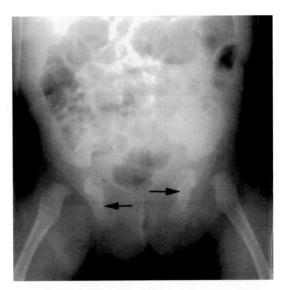

Figure 13–6. Bony changes of exstrophy of the bladder. Note that the region of the symphysis pubis is widened markedly *(arrows)*.

there is excessive widening of the symphysis pubis (Fig. 13–6). Normal width of the symphysis pubis is 1 centimeter no matter the age of the patient.

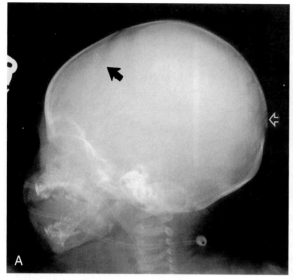
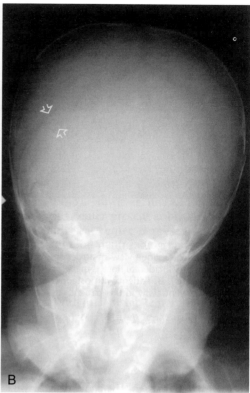
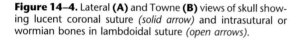

Figure 14–4. Lateral **(A)** and Towne **(B)** views of skull showing lucent coronal suture *(solid arrow)* and intrasutural or wormian bones in lambdoidal suture *(open arrows)*.

elements are incompletely ossified, particularly the spinous processes (Fig. 14–5). This fact allows spinal cord ultrasound to be done easily in the neonatal period, since the ultrasound beam can pass through the cartilaginous posterior elements.

On the lateral view of the vertebral bodies, there is usually a physiologic thoracolumbar kyphosis that resolves once axial loading occurs. In the vertebral body itself, there is sometimes a vertical radiolucency present that is called a coronal cleft (Fig. 14–6). This represents a notochordal remnant that is frequently seen in the lumbar spine and is more commonly present in males than females. It ossifies gradually in infancy and may leave a sclerotic area in the middle of the vertebral body. Coronal clefts can also be seen in a type of neonatal dwarfism called chondrodysplasia punctata, the rhizomelic form.

THORACIC CAGE

On the normal neonatal chest there are 12 pairs of ribs. If there are only 11 pairs of ribs, Down syndrome may exist. If there are more than 12 pairs present, the VACTERL association may be represented. The thoracic cage should not have a bell-shaped appearance at birth. When present, three separate causes should be considered. First, the hypotonic infant such as one with Down syndrome (Fig. 1–5, 5–3C, 5–7, 7–4) will have the most striking bell-shaped thoraces of all hypotonic infants. Second, iatrogenic sedation of the infant, either from maternal sedation or other sedation will cause a bell-shaped thorax. Once the sedation wears off, the chest will no longer be bell shaped. Third, hypoplastic lungs cause the bell shape because there is not enough aerated lung to keep the thoracic cage a normal shape. Clinically, this entity should be obvious if it is severe; a history of maternal oligohydramnios might be obtained.

On the lateral view the ossification centers for the manubrium and sternum should be assessed. There is usually one manubrial ossification center, which is separate from the sternal centers. There can be up to seven centers for the sternum (Fig. 14–7). If there are two manubrial ossification centers present, Down syndrome should be excluded, because this finding is present in 90 percent of

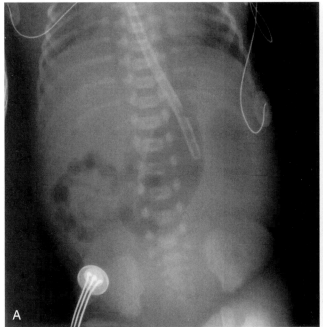

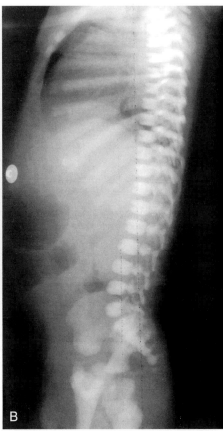

Figure 14–5. Frontal view **(A)** showing lumbar spine in a neonate where there is no ossification of the spinous processes. Incidental note of bowel obstruction is made. Lateral view **(B)** showing a normal thoracolumbar spine of another neonate.

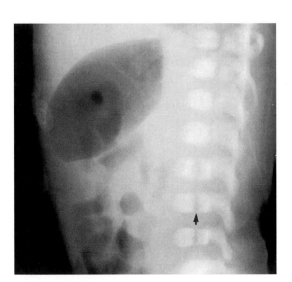

Figure 14–6. Lateral view of lumbar spine in male infant showing coronal clefts *(arrow)*, a normal variant.

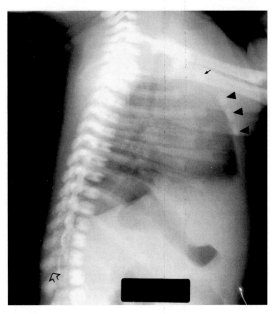

Figure 14–7. Lateral view showing normal sternal *(arrowheads)* and manubrial *(black arrow)* ossification centers that are distinctly separated. Patient also has punctate calcifications around posterior elements of spine due to maternal warfarin therapy *(open arrow)*.

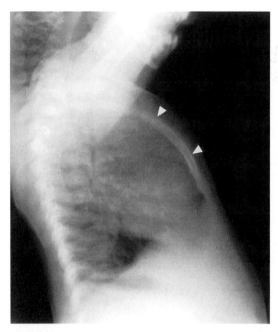

Figure 14–8. Patient with recombinant 8 syndrome showing no separation between the manubrial and sternal ossification centers *(arrowheads)*.

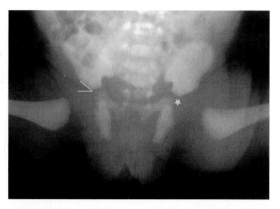

Figure 14–9. Anteroposterior view of the pelvis in a neonate showing the area of the triradiate cartilage *(star)* and the acetabular angle as demonstrated by the white lines.

PELVIS

The pelvis of the neonate shows lucencies between the pelvic bones due to the presence of cartilage. The most important of these cartilaginous areas is the triradiate cartilage from which the iliac, pubic, and ischial bones are attached and grow. This landmark is at the most medial aspect of the acetabulum. The acetabulum can be measured by drawing a line along its superiormost rim and intersecting it with a line drawn horizontally, but perpendicularly, to the triradiate cartilage. The angle is called the acetabular angle and is less than 30 degrees in the neonate (Fig. 14–9). Angles greater than this are associated with developmental dysplasia of the hip. Angles approaching zero may be associated with underlying skeletal dysplasias.

patients with this syndrome. If there is a lack of clear separation between the manubrial and sternal ossification centers, underlying congenital heart disease may be present. In addition, abnormal ossification of this area is seen with some chromosomal disorders such as trisomy 18 and recombinant 8 syndrome (Fig. 14–8), both of which have associated congenital heart disease as part of the chromosomal abnormality.

Chapter 15

The Neonate with Birth Trauma

CEPHALIC SOFT-TISSUE SWELLING

The head and extremities are the areas that chiefly experience trauma during a difficult delivery. Soft-tissue bruises seen clinically usually have no radiographic counterpart, except when the calvarium is involved. Soft-tissue calvarial swelling that crosses sutures is scalp edema, also known as caput succedaneum. Swelling that does not cross the sutures is called a cephalohematoma and represents a subperiosteal hematoma (Fig. 15–1). When the cephalohematoma resolves, it calcifies from the periphery inward and eventually becomes incorporated into the skull. The cephalohematoma is rarely associated with underlying skull fracture, although plain skull radio-graphs are frequently done to look for the fracture.

FRACTURES

Fractures can result from birth trauma. The calvicle is the most common fracture to be sustained from birth trauma (Fig. 15–2). Next, the humerus is most commonly fractured, followed by the femur. (In child abuse, the femur is the most commonly fractured long bone, followed by the tibia, and then followed by the humerus.) Rib fractures rarely result from birth trauma (Fig. 15–3). When healing rib fractures are encountered in the older neonate and infant, child abuse is most often the reason for the rib abnormality.

ERB PALSY

With shoulder dystocia, clavicle fractures are seen, and Erb palsy (nerve roots C5 through C7) can be diagnosed clinically. Radiographically, there is no finding present at birth, but there are findings in the older child. The shoulder becomes

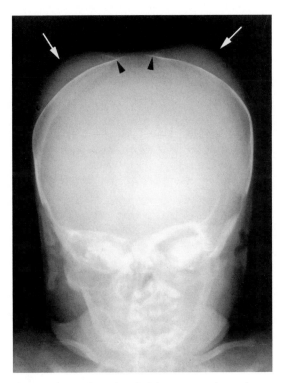

Figure 15–1. Bilateral cephalohematomas *(arrows)* stop at the sagittal suture and are beginning to calcify medially *(arrowheads).*

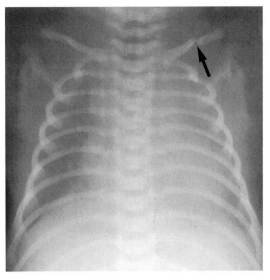

Figure 15–2. Fractured clavicle *(arrow)* from birth trauma is the most frequently encountered fracture.

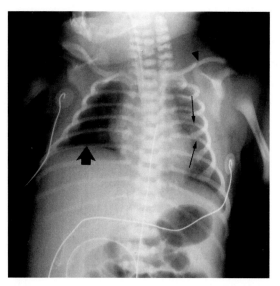

Figure 15-3. Birth trauma resulting in a fractured left clavicle *(arrowhead)* and paralyzed right hemidiaphragm *(large arrow)*. Note two left-sided rib fractures, as well *(small arrows)*.

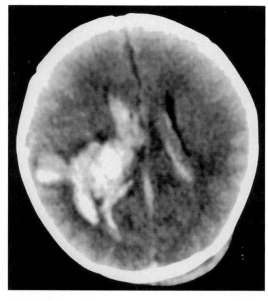

Figure 15-4. Patient's CT scan after vacuum extraction resulting in a massive intracranial hemorrhage. The white areas inside the calvarium represent acute hemorrhage.

dysplastic with age. Occasionally, the C4 nerve root is involved in this traumatic process, resulting in phrenic nerve palsy or paralysis. In these cases a plain chest radiograph can be used to suggest the diagnosis. The affected hemidiaphragm is uniformly elevated (Fig. 15–3). The hemidiaphragm may not be elevated in a patient who is being mechanically ventilated. At fluoroscopy or ultrasound, the hemidiaphragm shows paradoxical movement when not mechanically ventilated, which confirms the diagnosis. In general, patients who suffer from shoulder dystocia should be imaged with a chest radiograph to evaluate the clavicle and to investigate the possibility of hemidiaphragm abnormality.

INTRACRANIAL INJURY

Patients born with the assistance of the vacuum extractor device are at risk for intracranial hemorrhage (Fig. 15–4). These infants frequently present with seizures, which necessitates a lumbar puncture being performed on them. When the cerebrospinal fluid is bloody, unenhanced computed tomography (CT) of the head is the next imaging modality to determine the location and extent of intracranial hemorrhage. In the acute setting, magnetic resonance imaging (MRI) is not indicated. If the neonate's neurological examination is abnormal later, the MRI is the procedure of choice for assessing brain parenchymal damage.

Chapter 16

The Neonate with Loose Hips on Physical Examination

DEVELOPMENTAL DYSPLASIA OF THE HIP

Developmental dysplasia of the hip (DDH), formerly known as congenital dysplasia of the hip, is more commonly seen in girls, with the left side more often affected. Etiology is related to in utero positioning and ligamentous laxity as a result of maternal hormonal stimulation or familial ligamentous laxity. DDH is a spectrum of hip abnormality ranging from frank dislocation, at the worst, to posterior placement (subluxation) in the joint but not dislocation, at best.

When DDH is suspected clinically, imaging should not be obtained until approximately 4 to 6 weeks following birth to allow for the maternal hormonal influence to wear off. The modality of choice for imaging DDH is hip ultrasound. It involves no radiation, it can observe the hip in motion, and it can be done at the bedside. With plain film radiography, radiation is involved. This is an especially important consideration in girls and the radiograph is a static image. In addition, the ossified femoral head is usually not apparent radiographically and the location of the cartilaginous femoral head can only be inferred by plain

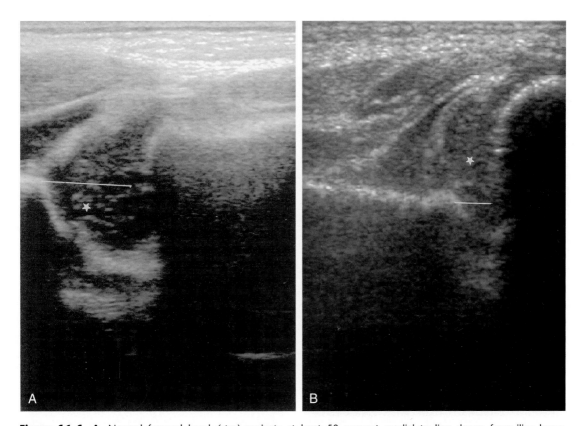

Figure 16–1. A, Normal femoral head *(star)* projects at least 50 percent medial to line drawn from iliac bone. **B,** Dislocated. Femoral head projects lateral and superior to acetabulum, as demarcated by the white line.

film radiography. Usually on ultrasound, the cartilaginous head is easily seen. It is the ossification center of the femoral head that limits the ultrasound by blocking the ultrasound beam. Therefore, in the older infant, pelvic radiographs in both frontal projection and frog-leg projection are the images of choice. The frontal view is best for determining hip position, and the frog-leg lateral is the best for evaluating potential relocation of the hip if it was dislocated on the neutral frontal film. But in the neonate, hip ultrasound is the imaging modality of choice.

Ultrasound Imaging

The findings on ultrasound involve transverse and longitudinal images of the hip with the transducer located along the lateral aspect of the hip. In the longitudinal plane, the femoral head is related to the ileum. The longitudinal view is where the diagnosis of frank dislocation of the femoral head can be made. A line drawn parallel to the iliac bone should intersect the femoral head with the head projecting at least 50 percent medial to the iliac line (Fig. 16–1). The appearance of the acetabulum can also be assessed in this view.

The transverse view or axial view is the one where the diagnosis of hip loosening (subluxation) can be made. The femoral head should sit in the acetabulum, as a golf ball on a golf tee (Fig. 16–2). When the femoral head is subluxed, it migrates posteriorly toward the ischial component of the acetabulum.

Plain Film Radiography

On plain radiograph, if the ossific nucleus is not present, the position of the femoral head can be projected by drawing imaginary lines in a horizontal plane perpendicular to the triradiate cartilage (Hilgenreiner line) and a perpendicular line from the lateral aspect of the acetabulum (Perkins line) such that they intersect to form four quadrants with the femoral head mainly projecting in the lower inner quadrant (Fig. 16–3). Dislocation projects the unossified femoral head outside of the lower, inner quadrant and in the upper, outer quadrant. Acetabular dysplasia is usually seen as well with an increased acetabular angle identified (Fig. 16–4). In the older infant, delay in ossification of the femoral head is noted when compared to the normal side.

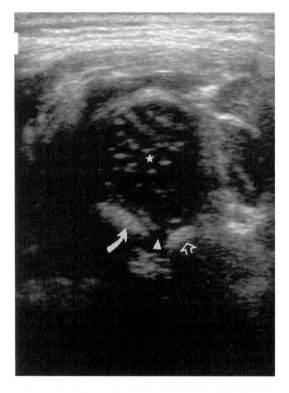

Figure 16–2. Femoral head *(star)* on axial view "sitting" on the "golf tee" made of the posterior ischial bone *(curved arrow)* and the anterior pubic bone *(open arrow)*. The triradiate cartilage is between *(arrowhead)*.

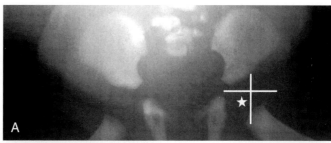

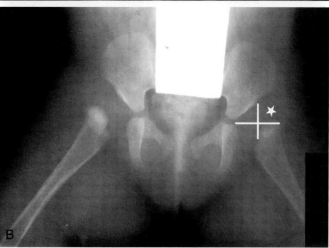

Figure 16–3. A, Normal. The unossified femoral head *(star)* projects in the lower inner quadrant made by the two lines, Hilgenreiner and Perkins. Note the abnormal sacral ossification centers. **B,** Dislocated. The unossified femoral head *(star)* projects in the upper outer quadrant in the dislocated hip.

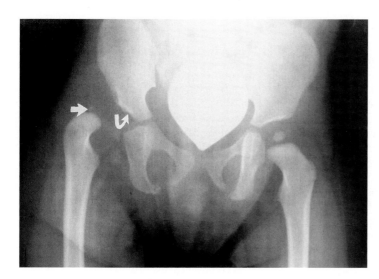

Figure 16–4. The dislocated hip on the right shows a small ossific nucleus *(arrow)* of the femoral head compared to the left and a dysplastic acetabulum *(curved arrow).*

Chapter 17

The Neonate with Dwarfism

Reference books on syndromes are a must, since there are so many skeletal dysplasias. However, some of the more common dysplasias can be readily diagnosed from plain radiographs. To evaluate the neonate for skeletal dysplasia completely, a skeletal survey must be obtained that includes frontal and lateral views of the spine and trunk, frontal views of the extremities, and three views of the skull. The most important views are the pelvis and lateral view of the spine.

Dwarfisms can be classified according to what part of the extremity is shortened. For example, rhizomelic dwarfism means that the "root" of the extremity is foreshortened (i.e., the humerus and femur). Mesomelic dwarfism means that the midportion of the extremity is foreshortened (i.e., radius and ulna and tibia and fibula). Some features of these dysplasias will be discussed.

ACHONDROPLASIA

Achondroplasia is the most common type of rhizomelic dwarfism. Most of the actors in *The Wizard of Oz* had this type of dwarfism. The hallmark of the diagnosis is narrowing of the interpediculate distance of the lumbar spine in the frontal view. This is the transverse distance between pedicles on the anteroposterior view. (Normally, this distance widens as one proceeds inferiorly in the lumbar spine [Fig. 17–1]). In addition, the proximal femoral metaphyses demonstrate an oval radiolucency because this area is narrowed from front to back. The pelvis has an unusual appearance in that the acetabular angles are flattened and the iliac wings have the appearance of tombstones. The sacrosciatic notch is small, and the appearance of the pelvic inlet has been compared to a champagne glass. The hands have shortened fingers that are all of the same length. The vertebral bodies are bullet-shaped on the lateral view, and there is frontal bossing on the lateral skull. The chest is somewhat narrowed. Later in life, these patients can suffer from hydrocephalus, because the calvarium has a small foramen magnum. In addition, spinal stenosis also becomes a problem due to the foreshort-

ened pedicles in the anterior-posterior dimension.

ASPHYXIATING THORACIC DYSTROPHY

Asphyxiating thoracic dystrophy, Jeune syndrome, is characterized by an extremely narrow chest with small lungs. An example of this syndrome is seen in Chapter 5 (Fig. 5–3B). As the name implies, patients can die from the respiratory complications of this dwarfism in the neonatal period, but not all of them do. The clavicles project high and have been compared to handlebars on a bicycle. It is also associated with renal abnormalities. There is frequently polydactyly, involving both the hands and feet. The pelvis is unusual with flattened acetabular angles. The configuration of the pelvic inlet has been compared to a wineglass. The capital femoral epiphysis is frequently ossified at birth. (Normally it is not present until 6 months of age.)

CHONDROECTODERMAL DYSPLASIA

A difficult distinction to make is to distinguish Jeune syndrome from chondroectodermal dysplasia, Ellis-van Creveld (EVC). In both these entities the thoraces are long and narrowed. In EVC there is no renal disease, but 50 percent of patients have congenital heart disease, frequently an atrial septal defect. In both entities there is polydactyly, although usually only in the hands with EVC. In the pelvis of patients with EVC, there is usually a bony spur projecting from the roof of the acetabulum medially, which is fairly characteristic of this disorder. This type of dwarfism is especially common in the Amish of Lancaster, Pennsylvania.

OSTEOGENESIS IMPERFECTA

When the bones are not sclerotic at birth and fractures are seen on neonatal radiographs, osteogenesis imperfecta (OI) should be diagnosed relatively easily. Clinically, these patients can have blue sclera, deafness, and sometimes abnormal dentition. In addition to the osteopenic bones

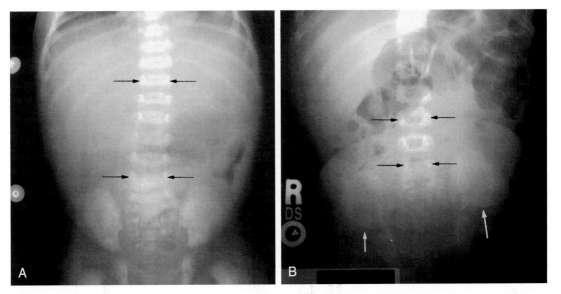

Figure 17–1. A, Normal frontal view of the lumbar spine where the interpediculate distance *(arrows)* widens as one proceeds inferiorly. **B,** Achondroplasia: the interpediculate distance narrows in the lumbar spine *(black arrows)* and the iliac wings have the appearance of tombstones with flattened acetabular angles *(white arrows)*.

radiographically, there are wormian bones (intrasutural bones) seen mainly in the lambdoid suture. Osteogenesis imperfecta originally was divided into two types, congenita and tarda. The congenita form was seen at birth, and the tarda form was seen later. Now this condition is more commonly divided into four types.

Type 1 is seen in childhood with osteopenic bones and fractures. The patients usually have blue sclera, deafness, and may also have abnormal dentition. Type 2 (Fig. 17–2) is the lethal form and previously was the congenita type of OI. The fractures are readily observed on prenatal ultrasound. The skeleton is profoundly osteopenic and gives no support to the soft-tissue structures. Patients afflicted with this type are frequently stillborn or die shortly after birth. Type 3 is less severe than type 2, but fractures can be present at birth. There is progressive deformity of the limbs into adulthood. Type 4 is the least severe of all the types and is difficult to diagnose initially. These patients usually do not have blue sclera or deafness. However, they eventually demonstrate osteopenia and may have femoral bowing. This mild form is rare.

THANATOPHORIC DWARFISM

Thanatophoric dwarfism ("death seeking") is easily diagnosed by the wafer-thin vertebral bod-

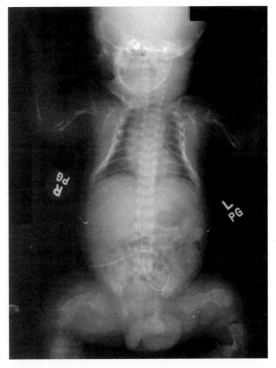

Figure 17–2. Osteogenesis imperfecta, type 2, formerly known as the congenita type. The bones are osteopenic and bowed from previous and current fractures.

ies that give them the appearance of a capital **H** on the frontal radiograph (Fig. 17–3). The femurs are short and bowed, which gives them the appearance of telephone receivers. The extremities, in general, are short (micromelic). The chest is narrow with short ribs. All affected infants are stillborn or die within a few hours of birth. Some patients can be born with premature cranial suture closure involving all sutures but the squamosal suture. This finding gives the calvarium a cloverleaf appearance.

EPIPHYSEAL CALCIFICATION DISORDERS

If punctate calcifications are seen in the region of the epiphyses, there are at least four diagnoses that can be suggested in the neonatal period. They are congenital stippled epiphyses (chondrodysplasia punctata), coumadin embryopathy, cerebrohepatorenal syndrome (Zellweger syndrome), and cretinism.

Chondrodysplasia Punctata

Chondrodysplasia punctata is a type of skeletal dysplasia that has two types—the severe, lethal

rhizomelic form, which is autosomal recessive, and the less severe form (Conradi-Hünermann) (Fig. 17–4), which is autosomal dominant. These two can be separated on the basis of the extreme rhizomelia and coronal clefts, which are seen in the first type. The patients with the rhizomelic form usually die of respiratory failure within the first year of life. It is important to see the neonatal films in order to make the diagnosis, because the punctate calcifications disappear after several months of life.

Coumadin Embryopathy

Coumadin embryopathy has the punctate calcifications (Fig. 14–7) but no rhizomelia. The bones otherwise look normal. There is associated midface hypoplasia.

Zellweger Syndrome

Zellweger syndrome characteristically has calcification in the region of the patella in the neonate (normal appearance time of patella ossification is around 3 years of age in girls). Again, there is no rhizomelia, but there is renal abnormality

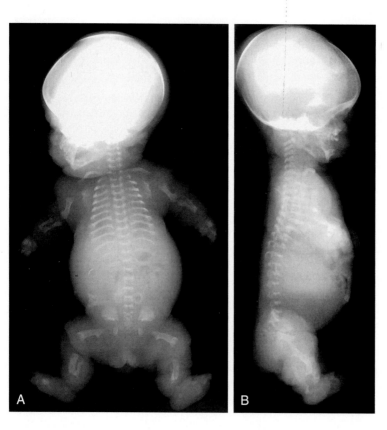

Figure 17–3. Frontal **(A)** and lateral **(B)** views of infant with thanatophoric dwarfism showing the extremely narrowed chest, short extremities, and wafer-thin vertebral bodies.

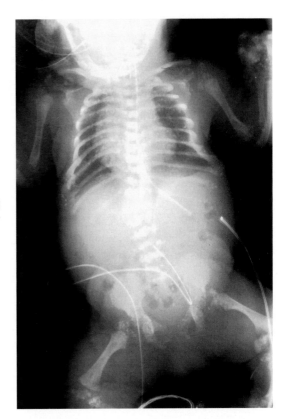

Figure 17–4. Chondrodysplasia punctata, the nonlethal form. Notice the stippled calcifications in all the cartilaginous areas.

(renal cysts) and brain dysgenesis (neuronal migrational disorders).

Cretinism

Cretinism causes delay in skeletal maturation, widened cranial sutures, and wormian bones as well as the stippled epiphyses. Again, there is no rhizomelia associated.

In general, the diagnosis of a skeletal dysplasia is not usually an emergency diagnosis. Just recognizing that there is something wrong with the bones and obtaining the appropriate skeletal survey is half the battle. Then a reference book on syndromes must be consulted. A dysmorphologist and pediatric radiologist familiar with skeletal dysplasias can be relied on to achieve the final diagnosis.

Chapter 18

The Neonate with Abnormal Bones Other than Skeletal Dysplasias

CONGENITAL INFECTIONS

Congenital infections can be associated with osseous abnormalities. The infections most commonly causing bony changes at birth are rubella, syphilis, and CMV (cytomegalic inclusion virus). CMV and rubella cause similar changes, but rubella causes delay in skeletal maturation such that the distal femoral epiphyseal and proximal tibial epiphyseal ossification centers are not present in the affected full-term infant (Fig. 18–1). Both infections can cause streaky lucencies in the metaphyses ("celery stalking"). Congenital syphilis causes diaphyseal periosteal new bone formation in the neonatal period as well as metaphyseal lucencies and metaphyseal erosions (Wimberger sign). All these infections usually are associated with hepatosplenomegaly, and CMV in particular is associated with intracranial calcifications.

ARTHROGRYPOSIS MULTIPLEX CONGENITA

Arthrogryposis multiplex congenita (AMC) is seen in neonates who do not move normally in utero but who are otherwise normal. They can be born with joint dislocations and contractures. Frequently seen abnormalities are developmental dysplasia of the hip, clubfeet, dislocated radial head, and decreased muscle mass with thin, osteopenic bones. Any neuromuscular disorder can cause thin bones, decreased muscle mass, and osteopenia but not the joint abnormalities seen with AMC. Other associated abnormalities seen in infants with neuromuscular abnormalities are bell-shaped thorax, which is due to the hypotonia, and tall vertebral bodies (Fig. 18–2).

TRISOMY 21 AND TRISOMY 18

Infants with trisomy 21 or trisomy 18, the most common trisomies, have associated bony abnor-

malities. Trisomy 21, as mentioned in other chapters, can be diagnosed radiographically by the presence of a bell-shaped chest, 11 pairs of ribs, double manubrial ossification center, and "Mickey Mouse" pelvis where the iliac bones are seen more *en face* and the acetabular angle is smaller than usual (Fig. 18–3). There is also a prominent right atrium seen on the chest radiograph regardless of the presence or absence of congenital heart disease. Trisomy 18, as described in Chapter 1, is associated with a dysplastic sternum seen on lateral chest radiograph (Fig. 1–7), long, thin ribs and clavicles (Fig. 1–3), and congenital vertical talus ("rocker-bottom" foot deformity). The iliac bones are also somewhat dysplastic, but this finding can be difficult to recognize.

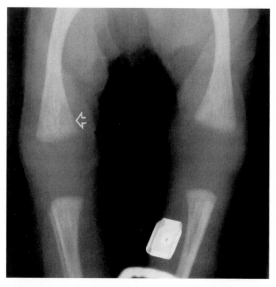

Figure 18–1. Congenital rubella, which causes the vertical striations *(arrow)* in the metaphyses ("celery stalking") and delay in skeletal maturation. This term infant should have distal femoral and proximal tibial ossification centers.

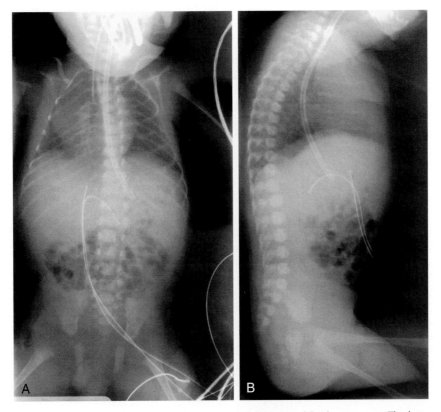

Figure 18–2. A, Frontal view of newborn with maternal history of decreased fetal movement. The bones are thin and osteopenic. Note the position of the two umbilical vein lines—one is stuck at the ductus venosus and the other is in the left portal vein. **B,** Lateral view showing the tall vertebral bodies in this patient with a neuromuscular disorder.

OSTEOPENIA

Nutrition is a difficult problem in the newborn intensive care unit, especially in the extremely premature infant. The sick neonates tend to get osteopenic just because they are not moving, usually because of heavy sedation. Others actually develop changes of rickets, although this problem is well recognized and is not as common today. The radiographic changes of rickets consist of osteopenia with loss of the white line at the end of the metaphysis (i.e., provisional zone of calcification), and if the rickets is not recognized, the metaphyses can become frayed. These acquired causes of osteopenia, both sedation and nutrition, can be associated with fractures. Those osteopenic infants requiring chest physiotherapy are at risk for rib fractures, which are frequently encountered (Fig. 18–4). However, rib fractures can also be seen in the absence of osteopenia as a result of repeated chest physiotherapy. Occasionally long bone fractures are seen as a result of the osteopenia.

OSTEOMYELITIS

Osteomyelitis can occur in the neonate. As in older children, the most common etiologic agent is staphylococcus. Osteomyelitis is most frequently a result of disseminated infection rather than a localized process. There is often associated septic arthritis. In the hip and shoulder, this process can be recognized radiographically by the femur or humerus being frankly dislocated (Fig. 18–5) or laterally displaced from the expected location in the joint. Bony changes take several days to develop and consist of a moth-eaten appearance to the involved bone (Fig. 18–6) with associated reparative new bone around it. Soft-tissue swelling can be seen before the bony counterparts occur. Nuclear medicine bone scan may be normal in neonates as opposed to older children and adults. The reason for this might be a different pathophysiology for osteomyelitis in the neonate or a suboptimal imaging technique with the normally "hot" physeal area masking the abnormal area of radioactivity. Since the infection

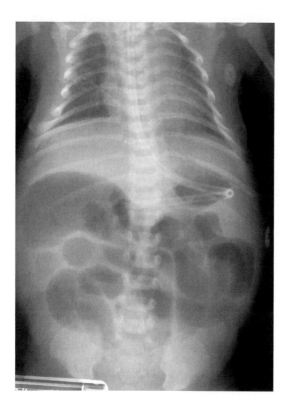

Figure 18–3. Trisomy 21 patient with bell-shaped chest and "Mickey Mouse ears" pelvis. Note the abnormal bowel gas pattern in this patient with long-segment Hirschsprung syndrome.

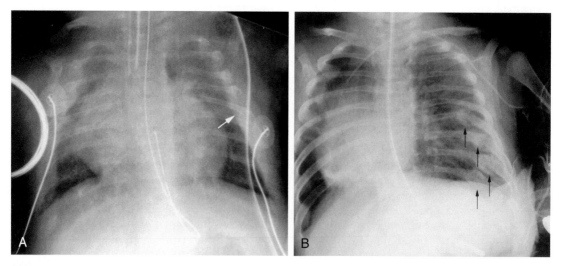

Figure 18–4. A, Patient with osteopenia from prolonged hospitalization and poor nutrition. Multiple rib fractures can be seen, especially laterally *(arrow)*. **B,** Patient in the hospital his entire life with rib fractures resulting from chest physiotherapy *(arrows)*.

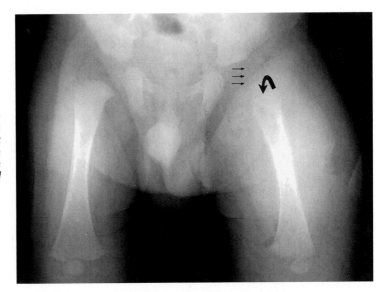

Figure 18–5. Patient with septic hip that led to osteomyelitis of the femoral shaft. The hip is dislocated *(straight arrows)*. There is diffuse swelling of the thigh, and there is destruction of the proximal femoral metaphysis *(curved arrow)*.

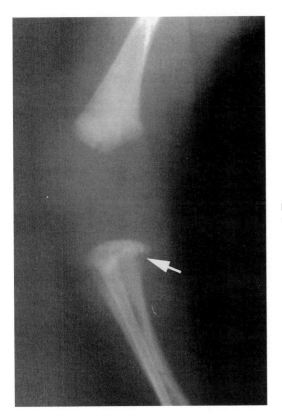

Figure 18–6. Premature infant with osteomyelitis of the proximal tibia as seen by the lytic lesion in the metaphysis *(arrow)*.

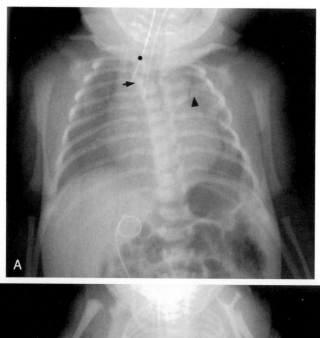

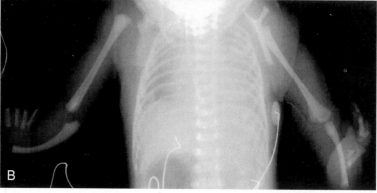

Figure 18–7. A, Patient with the VACTERL association. This patient has a hemivertebra of the upper thoracic spine *(arrow)*, which is associated with rib anomalies *(arrowhead)*. The patient is intubated, but the orogastric tube *(asterisk)* is stuck in the proximal pouch due to esophageal atresia and associated tracheoesophageal fistula. **B,** VACTERL association with radial ray anomaly bilaterally. Neither upper extremity has a radius or thumb. Patient also had imperforate anus and unilateral renal agenesis.

is frequently a manifestation of systemic infection, it is worthwhile to image the rest of the skeleton using bone scan or skeletal survey to diagnose multiple sites of potential involvement.

VACTERL ASSOCIATION

VACTERL association (V = vertebral abnormality, A = anal malformation, C = cardiac anomaly, TE = esophageal atresia with or without tracheoesophageal fistula, R = renal or rib deformity, and L = limb abnormality, especially radial ray anomaly) should be considered whenever there are vertebral anomalies (Fig. 18–7). These anomalies are sometimes best viewed on the first neonatal radiograph when there might not be that much abdominal gas to obscure the bony findings. The abnormalities can consist of a hemivertebra, a block-type vertebra where the two bodies are not completely separated, or other segmentation anomalies of the vertebral bodies. Specific types or sites of vertebral anomalies can suggest an underlying abnormality. For example, sacral abnormalities are frequently associated with imperforate anus, especially the high imperforate anus lesions.

Chapter 19

The Neonate with an Unusually Shaped Head

NORMAL SKULL

Evaluation of the abnormal skull must occur after learning what is a normal appearance to the calvarium in the neonate. The usual skull series consists of at least the frontal, one lateral, and the Towne view, which is an angled posterior view of the skull. The submentovertex view, which visualizes the calvarium inferiorly, can be included when there is concern of metopic synostosis.

There is usually a large ratio of the area in the calvarium when compared to the area in the face. This ratio is known as the craniofacial ratio. In the premature and term infant, this ratio is usually between 4 to 5:1 (Fig. 19–1). The adult ratio is approximately 2:1.

In the neonate the sutures are usually widely spread apart as a result of the molding that occurs in the birthing process. There are frequently skin folds causing artifacts in neonates due to such

redundant skin in these babies. Vascular markings are not seen in the neonate. Intrasutural bones or wormian bones may be seen in the lambdoidal suture in the neonate, although they are easier to see in the older infant and child. Sometimes there is a prominence to the occiput called bathrocephaly that usually disappears by 3 months with no sequelae. The paranasal sinuses are too underdeveloped to be seen in the neonate.

MOLDING FORCES

Most commonly, an unusually shaped head in the neonate is due to the molding that occurs with birth. The sutures are frequently overlapping, and there may be scalp edema (i.e., caput succedaneum) or subperiosteal hematoma (i.e., cephalohematoma). These findings resolve over several days. As the cephalohematoma resolves, the edges of it become firmer due to calcification and eventually it is incorporated into the calvarium. Plain

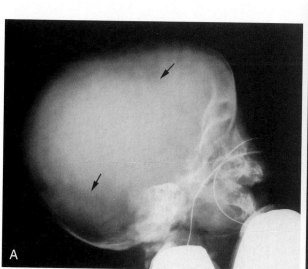 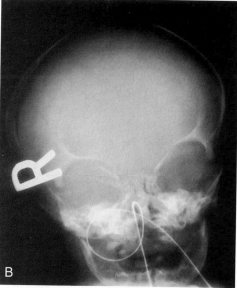

Figure 19–1. A, Lateral skull of premature infant showing the normal craniofacial ratio and wide-open sutures *(arrows).*
B, Normal frontal view of the same infant's skull.

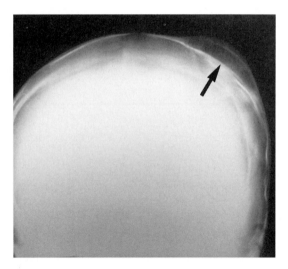

Figure 19–2. Calcified cephalohematoma *(arrow)* that will eventually become incorporated in the calvarium.

skull radiographs usually show a circular pattern to the calcification when seen *en face* and a rounded, moundlike appearance when seen tangentially (Fig. 19–2).

An unusually shaped head may also be due to positional forces. Premature neonates who constantly have their heads positioned on one side or the other usually will eventually demonstrate an elongated skull. Because of the new Sudden Infant Death Syndrome (SIDS) Prevention Guidelines advising against prone sleeping of infants, there is much more positional flattening seen in the occipital region in infants.

CRANIOSYNOSTOSIS

Craniosynostosis can also cause an unusually shaped head. Craniosynostosis is defined as the calvarial sutures fusing prematurely. Imaging of the sutures is best achieved by skull radiographs in the frontal, lateral, Towne, and submentovertex positions. When there is craniosynostosis present, the calvarium can no longer grow perpendicular to the suture. Instead, growth of the skull is achieved in a direction parallel to the suture. Radiographically, the suture has the appearance of being totally obliterated or is sclerotic along its margins with a "heaped-up" appearance to the edges.

The suture most commonly prematurely fused is the sagittal suture. This fusion causes the calvarium to elongate, resulting in an appearance called scaphocephaly or dolichocephaly (Fig. 19–3). The elongation is best seen on the lateral view, but the actual suture fusion is seen either on the Towne view or the frontal view. When the entire coronal suture is synostosed, the calvarium is foreshortened, which is known as brachycephaly. The orbits also are unusual in appearance with coronal synostosis in that they have the appearance of a "harlequin eye." If there is only unilateral synostosis, then just the ipsilateral orbit takes on the harlequin-eye appearance (Fig. 19–4). (Neonates tend to normally have orbits that resemble the harlequin-eye shape, but a search for the coronal suture reveals that it is not synostosed.) The coronal suture is best seen on the lateral view, which is the view to see the brachycephaly, but

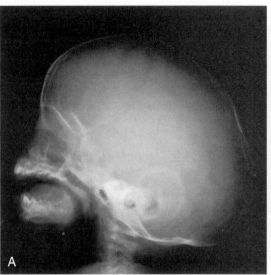
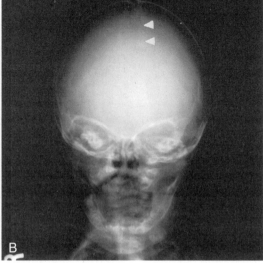

Figure 19–3. A, Lateral view showing an elongated skull in a patient with sagittal synostosis. **B,** Frontal view showing sclerosis *(arrowheads)* of the sagittal suture.

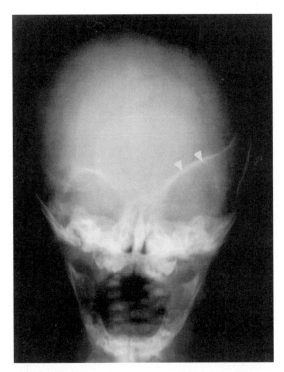

Figure 19–4. Unilateral coronal synostosis resulting in a unilateral "harlequin-eye" *(arrowheads)* appearance to the orbit.

the harlequin eye is best seen on the frontal image.

Other synostosed sutures that are much less common include the lambdoid suture that causes the skull to be flattened posteriorly on the involved side if unilateral involvement occurs. This is called plagiocephaly. This suture is best evaluated on the Towne view. When the metopic suture is prematurely fused, the calvarium has a ridge in the frontal portion (trigonocephaly) and the orbits have an appearance of being angled upward medially. The frontal ridge is best appreciated on the submentovertex view and the orbital appearance is seen on the frontal view.

Other imaging modalities, bone scanning and CT, have been studied in the literature to evaluate for craniosynostosis. Nuclear medicine bone scanning was initially used for this evaluation based on the theory that normal, nonfused, sutures are metabolically active and show increased radiopharmaceutical uptake, whereas fused sutures do not. However, there is such slow bone turnover in the calvarium that it is hard to tell metabolically inactive sutures from normal ones. In addition, bone scanning is much more expensive than skull radiographs. Also there is no sedation involved with skull x-rays as there usually is in nuclear medicine imaging. On the other hand, CT scanning of the calvarium is almost too sensitive for this evaluation, in that the suture can frequently be seen on CT scan and the appearance may simulate that the suture is still open when it really is functionally closed. CT scanning can be performed to evaluate any potential underlying brain malformations, but this is an expensive procedure with a low yield since there is almost no association of underlying brain abnormalities with craniosynostosis.

Chapter 20

The Newborn Infant with a Small Head Circumference, Drop in Hematocrit, or Change in Neurologic Status

A small head circumference in a neonate is worrisome for underlying brain parenchymal abnormalities, because it is brain growth that causes the calvarium to grow. Congenital infections and brain malformations are two reasons for small measurements of the head circumference.

ULTRASOUND IMAGING

Ultrasound is an excellent screening modality for these problems, since it is portable, quick, relatively inexpensive, and involves no radiation. The transducer is placed on the anterior fontanel, which stays open for several months. (Other investigators have also used the thin temporal bone, the orbit, the posterior fontanel when present, and the foramen magnum as "windows" to visualize the brain.) Images through the anterior fontanel are obtained in both the coronal and sagittal planes. These planes are angled and the anatomy is not seen in the same way as if the planes were obtained in direct coronal and sagittal planes as they are with MRI and CT. If an underlying brain malformation is seen on ultrasound, then other imaging modalities such as CT or MRI can be obtained for confirmation of a suspected disorder.

Normal head ultrasound in the premature infant shows the brain to be relatively homogeneous in echogenicity because of the presence of little sulcation, especially in the extremely premature infant (Fig. 20–1). The ventricles are slightly more prominent, as is the choroid plexus in the premature infant when compared to the term brain. There may be slight ventricular asymmetry, but this is a normal finding. The choroid plexus is usually symmetric and echogenic in appearance. As in all of radiology, abnormal findings must be confirmed on two views at 90 degrees to one another (i.e., sagittal and coronal images).

CONGENITAL INFECTIONS

The most common congenital infections to cause cerebral problems are cytomegalic inclusion virus (CMV) and toxoplasmosis. Congenital rubella is rarely seen today. All are associated with microcephaly. CMV and toxoplasmosis both cause intracranial calcifications that can be indistinguishable in their pattern of calcification. Characteristically, CMV causes calcification in a periventricular distribution and toxoplasmosis causes more of a parenchymal distribution of calcification. Congenital inflections can also cause echogenic vessels in the thalamus (Fig. 20–2). If CMV is present at the time of organogenesis, serious malformations of the brain can result. Usually, the CMV destroys brain, which results in loss of brain parenchyma and ventricular dilatation that fills in the space that was supposed to be normal brain. CMV is more commonly seen than toxoplasmosis. Ultrasound is usually the first imaging modality employed for microcephaly, but a CT scan is frequently performed to confirm questionable findings (Fig. 20–3).

BRAIN MALFORMATIONS

Agenesis of Corpus Callosum

Midline abnormalities such as agenesis of the corpus callosum (CC) are readily seen on ultrasound. The sagittal midline image in the normal infant shows a relatively hypoechoic corpus callosum with sulcation that parallels the CC (Fig. 20–4). When the CC is absent, the sulcation radiates out like the spokes of a wheel around the area where the CC was supposed to be present (Fig. 20–5). When there is agenesis of the CC, there is also occipital horn dilatation called colpocephaly.

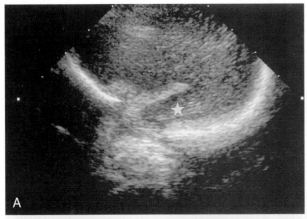

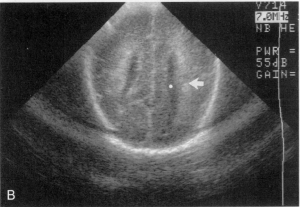

Figure 20–1. A, Sagittal image of an extremely premature infant showing a homogeneous echogenicity to the brain. (Temporal lobe is shown by the "star.") **B,** Coronal image of a premature brain showing the lateral ventricles *(asterisk)* and the normal periventricular hyperechogenicity *(arrow)*. Sulcation as seen by echogenic lines is almost absent due to the extreme prematurity of the infant. **C,** Sagittal image of a premature brain showing slight enlargement of the lateral ventricle *(asterisk)* due to previous hemorrhage that has resolved. The brain is homogeneously echoic. The choroid plexus is echogenic *(arrow)*.

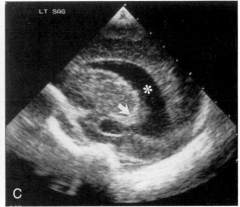

Absence of Septum Pellucidum

Absence of the septum pellucidum causes the appearance of a single, continuous frontal horn on coronal images. Its absence is not a normal variant and is most commonly a manifestation of a constellation of abnormalities called septooptic dysplasia (SOD) (Fig. 20–6). Associated with SOD are optic nerve atrophy and endocrine abnormalities due to pituitary problems. Some authors classify this dysplasia as the least severe type of holoprosencephaly.

Holoprosencephaly

Holoprosencephaly is defined by the presence of brain extending across the midline at some point. The most severe type is alobar (Fig. 20–7A) where there is no midline dividing point and a single large ventricle with fused thalami is seen. More midline division is seen with the semilobar and lobar types (Fig. 20–7B). MRI is helpful to diagnose the less severe types, although it is not necessary for the alobar types. The alobar type can be associated with trisomy 13 and is usually a fatal brain disorder. Clinically, the facial features of alobar holoprosencephaly are distinctive with midline cleft lip, hypotelorism, and a flat nasal bridge.

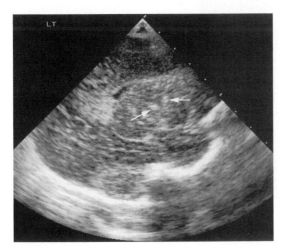

Figure 20–2. Neonate with echogenic vessels in the thalamus *(arrows)* due to CMV infection.

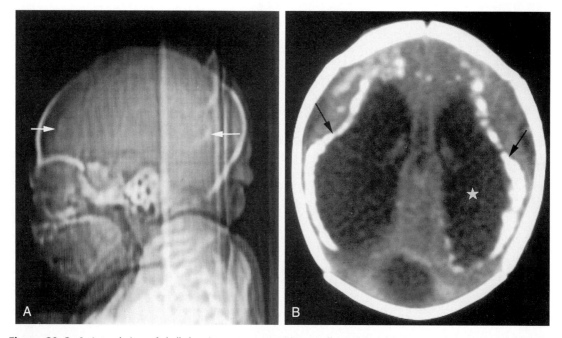

Figure 20–3. A, Lateral view of skull showing a neonate with a small craniofacial ratio as a result of congenital CMV. The periventricular calcifications are faintly seen *(arrows).* **B,** CT scan showing enlarged ventricles *(asterisk)* and periventricular and parenchymal calcifications *(arrows).*

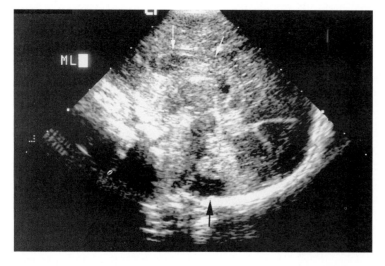

Figure 20–4. Normal midline structures in the sagittal plane. The corpus callosum is the hypoechoic C-shaped structure *(white arrows).* The cisterna magna is present below the vermis of the cerebellum *(black arrow).*

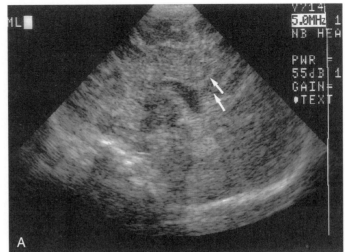

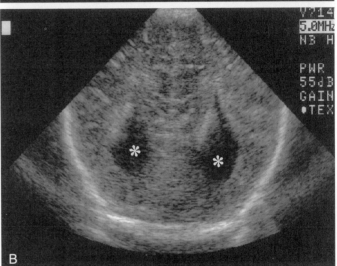

Figure 20–5. A, Midline sagittal image showing absence of the corpus callosum with the sulcation radiating out *(arrows)* like the spokes of a wheel. **B,** Abnormally dilated occipital horns of lateral ventricles *(asterisks)* in a patient with agenesis of the corpus callosum.

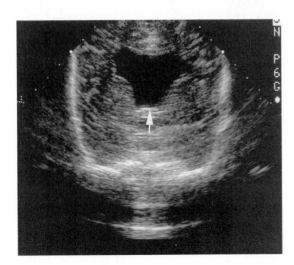

Figure 20–6. Absence of the septum pellucidum causes the frontal horns to become continuous. The arrow denotes where this structure should be.

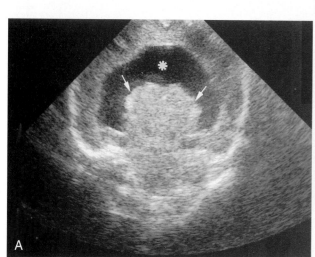
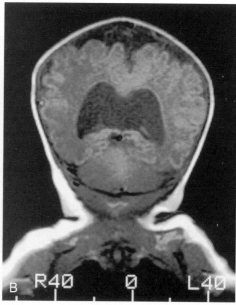

Figure 20–7. A, Alobar holoprosencephaly is shown by the monoventricle *(asterisk)* and fused thalami *(arrows).* **B,** MRI of a less severe holoprosencephaly, semilobar. Anterior to this image there was preservation of the midline.

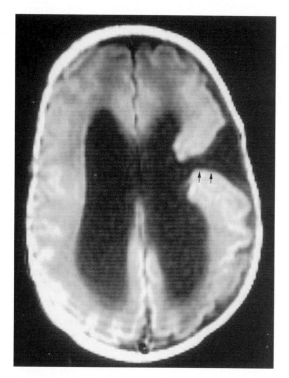

Figure 20–8. MRI of the brain showing schizencephaly, cleft in the brain. The cleft is lined by gray matter *(arrows).*

Schizencephaly

Schizencephaly is a cleft in the brain that communicates with the ventricle. The cleft is lined by gray matter, whereas an area of brain infarction (encephalomalacia) is not. There are two types: closed lip and open lip. In the closed lip type, the cleft is present but its communication with the ventricle can be subtle, since the gray matter on each side of the cleft is frequently touching. Ultrasound can visualize the cleft as a straight echogenic line extending from the ventricle to the brain surface. The open lip variety is much easier to see, since the cleft is widely spaced and filled with cerebrospinal fluid that communicates with the ventricle. Both of these types of schizencephaly are usually diagnosed on MRI (Fig. 20–8), because this imaging modality can visualize the gray matter lining the cleft better than other imaging methods.

INTRACRANIAL HEMORRHAGE AND HYPOXIC INJURY

Intracranial Hemorrhage

Postnatally, premature infants are particularly at risk for intracranial hemorrhage (ICH). The literature states that the incidence of ICH is from 25 percent to 40 percent, although this incidence may drop now that steroids are given to

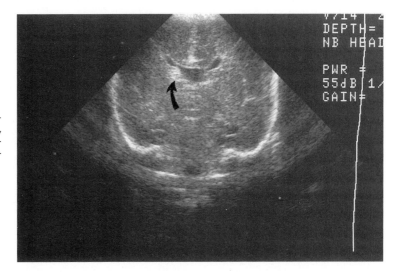

Figure 20–9. Patient with subependymal germinal matrix hemorrhage, grade 1 (arrow) with additional findings of absence of the septum pellucidum.

mothers prior to a premature delivery. In these infants, the subependymal germinal matrix is the region most sensitive to changes in oxygenation and blood pressure. It consists of a rich, vascular network of capillaries that have thin walls and can easily bleed. If the hemorrhage is confined to this region, it is called grade 1 (Fig. 20–9). If the hemorrhage breaks out into the ventricular lumen without ventricular dilatation, then the grade is 2. If there is associated ventricular dilatation at the time of initial diagnosis, then the grade is 3. If hemorrhage is seen in the parenchyma of the brain, then the grade is 4 (Fig. 20–10). Recent literature, however, supports the theory that the grade 4 hemorrhages are really periventricular venous infarctions. These infants are at greatest risk for hemorrhage in the first 3 to 4 days.

The first screening head ultrasound is usually performed at 5 to 7 days in prematures that are 32 weeks or less in gestational age. Follow-up examinations are performed weekly on those patients who have grade 2 or higher hemorrhages. In the case of grade 2, these examinations are to evaluate for ventricular dilatation and, in those cases of grade 3 or 4, to follow the already present ventricular dilatation. Discharge exams are performed on all infants with a birth weight of 1000 grams or less. Since the subependymal germinal matrix involutes by around 36 weeks of

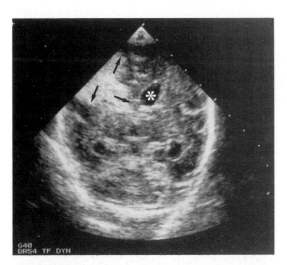

Figure 20–10. Slight ventricular dilation (asterisk) plus echogenicity in the right ventricle and into the parenchyma (arrows) is either a grade 4 intraventricular hemorrhage or a periventricular venous infarction.

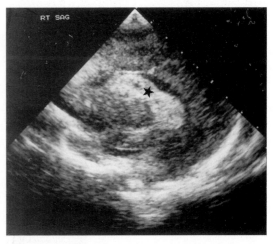

Figure 20–11. Sagittal image shows echogenicity (star) throughout the ventricle that is indistinguishable from choroid plexus. Time will help to make this distinction as the blood will become less echoic and the choroid will stay echogenic.

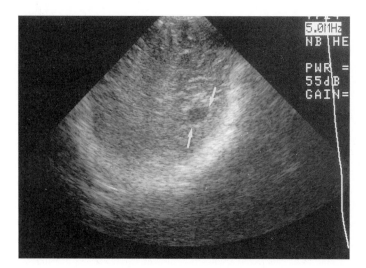

Figure 20–12. Hypoechoic hemorrhage *(arrows)* in this patient receiving extracorporeal membrane oxygenation who is systemically heparinized.

gestation, term infants that bleed do so in a different location than do premature infants. Usually these infants hemorrhage in the perichoroidal area with resultant intraventricular bleed. They can also bleed in the brain parenchyma, as well. The grading system only applies to premature infants.

Acute hemorrhage on ultrasound has an echogenic appearance, which then becomes less echoic and then hypoechoic before it is no longer appreciated on ultrasound. When the blood is acute in the ventricles, it can be difficult to distinguish from the normal choroid plexus (Fig. 20–11). Time helps to make this distinction. As the blood

becomes less echoic, the choroid stays the same. The location is also helpful in that there is no choroid plexus in the frontal horn or in the occipital horn. If there is increased echogenicity in these areas, hemorrhage must be assumed to be present. CT scan of the brain can be obtained to confirm these findings, if necessary, although this imaging method is rarely needed. Frequently, CT can't be performed because the infant is too unstable. An exception to this progression of hemorrhage appearance is in those patients that are on heparin for extracorporeal membrane oxygenation (ECMO) therapy. Since those patients cannot clot, the hemorrhage is initially hypoechoic (Fig.

Figure 20–13. This coronal image shows parenchymal echogenicity continuous with the ventricular lumen on the right *(straight arrow)*. On the left is patchy increased echogenicity that represents early periventricular leukomalacia *(curved arrow)*.

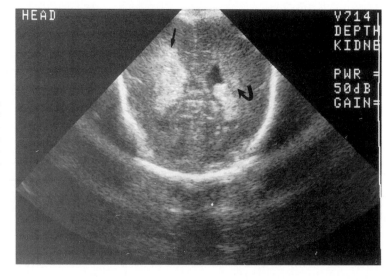

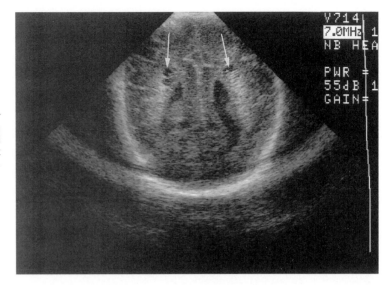

Figure 20–14. Cystic periventricular leukomalacia (PVL) *(arrows)* seen in this patient on the predischarge head ultrasound. The lucencies do not communicate with the ventricles, which is typical for PVL.

20–12). Once the anticoagulant is stopped, the hemorrhage becomes echogenic and then follows the usual sequence.

Periventricular Leukomalacia

Premature infants are also at risk for hypoxic changes to the brain other than intracranial hemorrhage. In the premature infant, the periventricular white matter is a watershed area and is the area of greatest risk for hypoxic damage. (Term infants have both white and gray matter injury in response to hypoxia.) These hypoxic changes tend to manifest in these areas, and the constellation of findings is called periventricular leukomalacia (PVL). Sonographically, PVL is echogenic initially because of parenchymal edema (Fig. 20–13). It can be extremely difficult to separate parenchymal hemorrhage from parenchymal edema. Again, location and time can help. PVL tends to be bilateral, although it may be asymmetric in appearance. In addition, if the edematous change proceeds to infarction with resultant encephalomalacia (which looks cystic on US), the cystic change usually does not communicate with the ventricle in PVL (Fig. 20–14) but does communi-

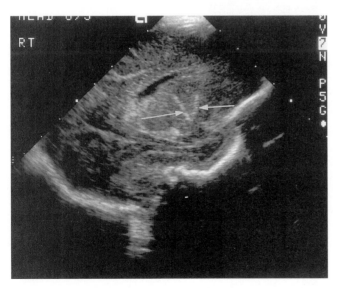

Figure 20–15. Abnormal vessels are clearly seen in this infant *(arrows)* in the thalamic region. No explanation for their appearance could be found.

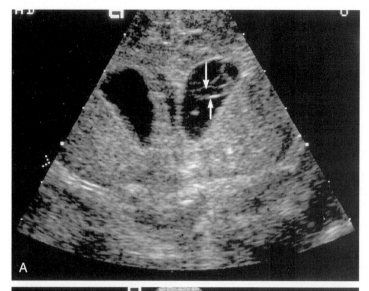

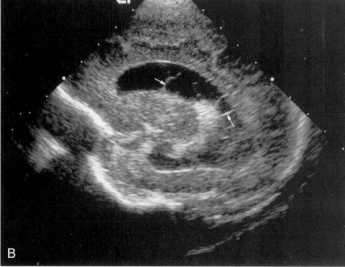

Figure 20–16. A, Coronal view. **B,** Sagittal view of patient suffering from ventriculitis due to *Escherichia coli* with resultant septation *(arrows)* in the ventricles and enlargement of the ventricles.

cate with the ventricle with parenchymal hemorrhage. This distinction is not always clear-cut, and there is an overlap of findings. Frequently, there is both PVL and intracranial hemorrhage present in the same infant.

Abnormal Vessels in the Thalamus

Other echogenic abnormalities in the brain of neonates include abnormal vessels in the region of the thalamus. The abnormal vessels (Fig. 20–15) can be seen in a variety of situations including hypoxia, maternal cocaine ingestion, chromosomal abnormalities such as trisomies, and congenital infections. The prognostic significance of this finding is unknown.

Ventriculitis

Infection in the ventricle, although uncommon, can result in the creation of septation and ventricular dilation (Fig. 20–16). These findings can be indistinguishable from previous intraventricular hemorrhage.

Chapter 21

The Neonate with Midline Back Abnormalities

On physical examination of the newborn infant, observation of the back is important for evaluation of possible midline abnormalities that can have neurologic sequelae associated with them. These midline back abnormalities are termed dysraphism or neural tube defects. When the dysraphism is open (spina bifida cystica), it is clinically obvious as a midline defect. These infants have neurologic abnormality at the outset. When it is closed (spina bifida occulta), there usually are only cutaneous manifestations such as a hairy nevus or deep sacral dimple. These patients are neurologically normal in the neonatal period.

SPINA BIFIDA CYSTICA

Spina bifida cystica most often includes either a myelomeningocele or myelocele. These patients also have Chiari II malformation that usually results in hydrocephalus. Sometimes the hydrocephalus does not become obvious until the neural tube defect is closed. Imaging of these infants includes plain radiographs to assess bony abnormalities associated with spina bifida. These changes include widening of the interpediculate distances with narrowing of the pedicles in the transverse plane (Fig. 21–1), lack of bony ossification of the posterior elements, and sometimes there are vertebral body fusion abnormalities. Plain skull radiographs, although unnecessary, demonstrate thinning of the calvarium in a patchy distribution, which is called lacunar skull (also called Lückenschädel). This appearance is not due to underlying increased intracranial pressure but is a developmental dysplasia of the bone that disappears around 6 to 9 months of age (Fig. 21–2).

Head ultrasound of these neonates is recommended for evaluating the degree of ventricular dilatation preoperatively so that the ventricles can be shunted at the time of the neural tube defect repair if they are large enough. Postoperative head ultrasound (Fig. 21–3) can be performed to evaluate shunt position and to observe for ventricular dilatation in those patients that don't initially require shunting prior to closure of the defect. Patients that have hydrocephalus, for whatever reason, usually will have the shunts placed into the right parietal region (nondominant hemisphere). Then there should be several centimeters of shunt placed in the peritoneal cavity to allow for growth of the patient. Incidentally, a shunt series is a frontal and lateral view of the entire shunt (Fig. 21–4). When shunt malfunction is suspected, an evaluation is made of the continuity of the shunt and the potential CSF pseudocyst in the abdomen that can result in shunt malfunction.

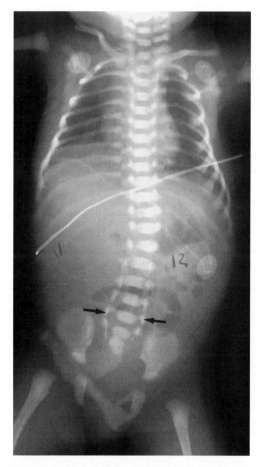

Figure 21–1. Patient with myelomeningocele with widening of the interpediculate distance and narrowing of the pedicles in the transverse plane *(arrows)*.

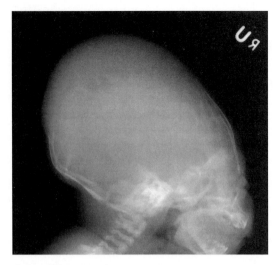

Figure 21–2. The calvarium in this newborn with Arnold-Chiari II malformation shows the irregular ossification of lacunar skull (i.e., Lückenschädel).

Spinal cord ultrasound can be performed postoperatively to evaluate associated spinal cord pathology (since there is no posterior element ossification to interfere with the ultrasound beam) such as diastematomyelia, hydromyelia, and tethering of the cord in the repair. However, most of the time these associated anomalies are evaluated by MRI.

A baseline renal ultrasound should also be obtained, because all patients with spina bifida have neurogenic bladders that can result in obstructed ureters or refluxing ureters with subsequent hydronephrosis. Renal anomalies also can be present. (Note: All patients that have neurogenic bladders need latex precautions instituted on them in the neonatal period.)

SPINA BIFIDA OCCULTA

Neonates that have midline back abnormalities such as a hairy nevus, bottomless sacral dimple, hemangioma, or other unusual midline marking should have a screening evaluation with ultrasound for cord abnormalities that can be associated with these cutaneous anomalies. (Patients with anorectal abnormalities also are at risk for spinal cord abnormalities and should be screened.) In this age group, the posterior elements of the vertebral column are not completely ossified, which allows the ultrasound beam to penetrate the cartilaginous elements with resultant visualization of the actual spinal cord. Plain lumbar spine radiographs are not necessary in this patient population (with the exception of those infants with anorectal malformations) and are usually of little value. The process of ossification is ongoing and is complete when a term infant is about 12 months of age. The spinous process ossification that occurs with time does interfere with the ultrasound evaluation, so the best time for ultrasound is within the first few months of life. After this time, spinal cord ultrasound is difficult, and MRI of the cord plays a larger role in screening for abnormalities.

The spinal cord is imaged in both the longitudinal and transverse planes with the infant in a prone position. The cord is relatively hypoechoic with an echogenic central echo complex (i.e., central canal). The canal usually is not seen as a fluid space but only as an echogenic dot (Fig. 21–5). A normal variant in the lumbar cord does demonstrate the canal as a small cerebrospinal fluid (CSF) space and is called the ventriculus terminalis (the "fifth" ventricle). Normally, the cord falls to the ventral portion of the canal in a prone

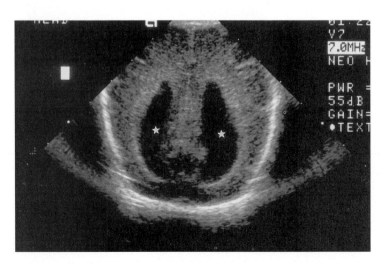

Figure 21–3. Postoperative patient with dilation of the occipital horns *(stars)* of the lateral ventricles but not large enough to need shunting.

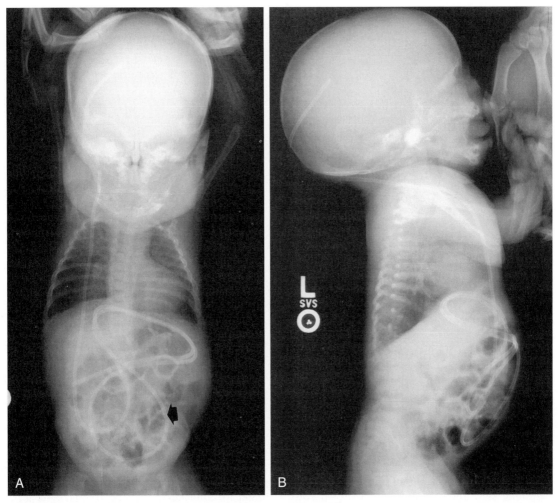

Figure 21–4. Shunt series frontal **(A)** and lateral **(B)** in a patient with posthemorrhagic hydrocephalus. Note the redundancy of the shunt in the abdomen *(arrow)* to allow for the growth of the child.

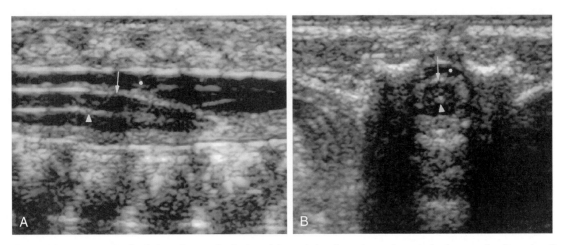

Figure 21–5. A, Longitudinal view of normal spinal cord *(arrow)* showing echogenic central echo complex *(arrowhead)* and dorsal subarachnoid space *(asterisk)*. **B,** Transverse view of normal spinal cord *(arrow)* showing echogenic central echo complex *(arrowhead)* and dorsal subarachnoid space *(asterisk)*.

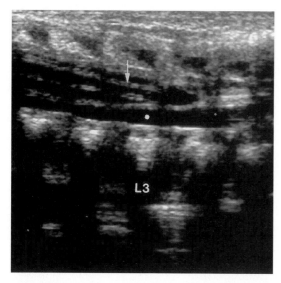

Figure 21–6. Tethered cord with the cord *(arrow)* ending below L3 vertebral body and preservation of the ventral subarachnoid space *(asterisk)*.

infant. In the longitudinal plane the level of the end of the cord (i.e., conus medullaris) is no lower than the superior endplate of L3 and frequently is at L2 or higher. The cord on the transverse images usually looks like a "target" with the hypoechoic cord surrounding the echogenic central echo complex. There are also intrinsic pulsations of the cord that can be difficult to see, particularly in the crying infant.

The most common pathology seen with the overlying skin abnormalities is a tethered cord with or without a mass, such as lipoma, to tether it. The hallmarks of a tethered cord are that the conus ends below L3 (Fig. 21–6) and the cord does not fall to the ventral portion of the canal but remains tacked up to the dorsal portion of the canal. Also the normal pulsations of the cord are lost and the filum terminale may be thickened. If tethered cord is suspected on ultrasound, then an MRI (Fig. 21–7) can be obtained within a few weeks for confirmation, if necessary. Surgery should soon follow to release the tethering so that the patient does not suffer neurologic sequelae as

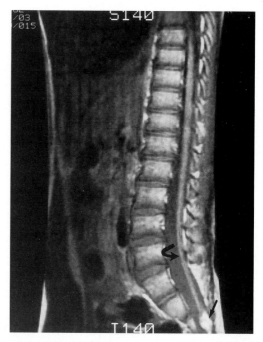

Figure 21–7. MRI of older child showing tethered cord *(curved arrow)* with lipoma at its caudal end *(straight arrow)*.

a result of the traction on the cord that can occur with growth of the infant.

Other than tethering of the cord, uncommon spinal cord pathology can be seen such as diastematomyelia (split cord) and hydromyelia (dilatation of the central canal). Diastematomyelia is diagnosed on ultrasound by the cord appearing wider than normal in the longitudinal view at the level where the division has taken place and then there are two distinct cords seen on the transverse view (two "targets"). At the site of the cord division, there is either a bony or cartilaginous spicule that tethers the cord at this site, which results in a neurologic abnormality in the patient's future if it is not released. The diagnosis of hydromyelia is made when there is abnormal dilation of the central echo complex such that the usual echogenic complex is seen as a CSF space. (This entity is not to be confused with the normal tiny CSF space known as ventriculus terminalis.)

Section II

The Older Infant and Child

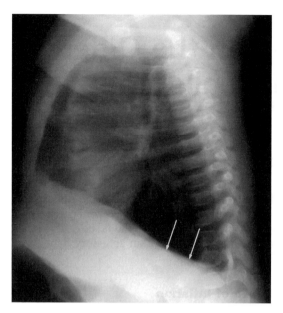

Figure 22–2. Lateral view of hyperinflated chest with flattening of the hemidiaphragms *(arrows)*.

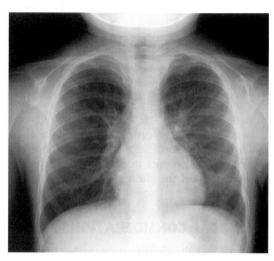

Figure 22–3. "Boxy" appearance to the thoracic cage indicative of chronic air trapping in this asthmatic patient.

no longer "domed"), then that patient is hyperinflated. With chronic air trapping the chest assumes a "boxy" appearance (Fig. 22–3).

TUBES AND LINES

Tubes and lines must also be visualized. Umbilical vessel catheters are no longer used, since the cord has long since dried up and fallen off. Most commonly, subclavian vein catheters and femoral vessel catheters are the mainstay of vascular access in older pediatric patients. A special type of venous line is a tiny, nearly radiolucent, percutaneous catheter with the flexibility of cooked spaghetti (Fig. 22–4). These catheters most commonly are inserted in the antecubital area and are threaded into the chest.

Endotracheal (ET) tubes again must be seen to project over the trachea somewhere between the carina and the thoracic inlet. In the older infant and child, the carina is usually easier to see, making assessment of the ET tube a little easier. However, without the aid of the lateral view it may be difficult to ascertain whether the tube is in the trachea versus the esophagus. ECG leads need to be moved, if possible, because they can obscure underlying pathology if the patient is small.

RIB CHANGES

The bony thorax should be scrutinized, since clues to underlying diagnoses can be obtained. Postthoracotomy rib changes usually consist of two ribs being closer together than the other ribs and frequently having a wavy contour (Fig. 22–5). The rib changes result when the surgeon ties the ribs together at the end of the thoracic surgical procedure. In the pediatric patient, right thoracotomy rib changes usually result from repair of esophageal atresia with or without tracheoesophageal fistula and palliative vascular shunts (most commonly Blalock-Taussig) in patients with congenital heart disease associated with right-sided obstructive lesions. Left thoracotomy rib changes usually result from great vessel surgeries such as patent ductus arteriosus ligation, coarctation repair, pulmonary artery banding, modified Blalock-Taussig shunts, and repair of esophageal atresia with or without tracheoesophageal fistula in those patients who have a right aortic arch. Median sternotomy wires are seen after repair of intracardiac shunts or complex congenital heart lesions.

Other rib changes that can be seen are rib fractures and rib notching. Since the thorax of the young child is elastic, rib fractures are encountered infrequently, even in the setting of massive

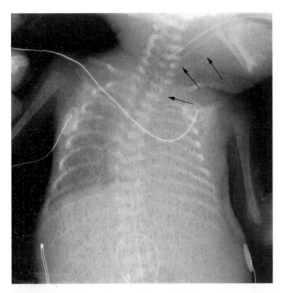

Figure 22–4. Small percutaneous lines are used in all age groups, including neonates. The catheters can be difficult to see and can end up in unusual places such as the neck *(arrows)*.

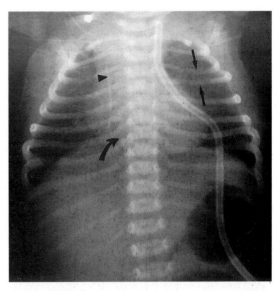

Figure 22–5. Left thoracotomy rib changes *(straight arrows)* for repair of esophageal atresia with tracheoesophageal fistula in patient with right aortic arch *(curved arrow)*. Percutaneous line *(arrowhead)* projects in the right atrium.

motor vehicle trauma. Therefore, when rib fractures are seen, child abuse must be suspected. Rib notching is present in patients with long-standing coarctation of the aorta and involves the inferior and lateral aspect of ribs three through eight (Fig. 22–6). The notching is a result of the dilated

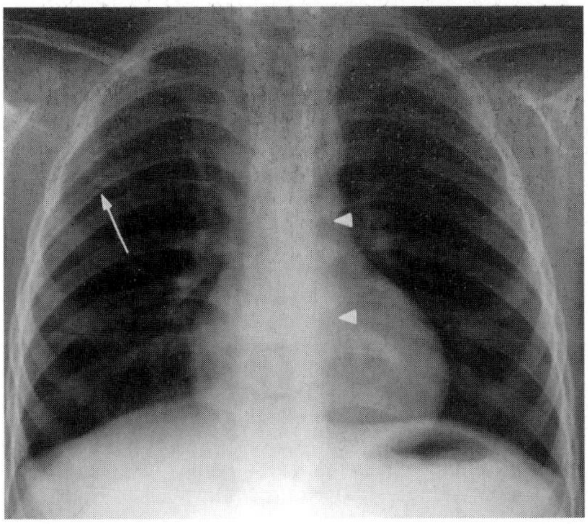

Figure 22–6. Frontal view of child with prominent descending thoracic aorta *(arrowheads)* due to coarctation. Subtle rib notching *(arrow)* can also be seen.

intercostal arteries that serve as collateral vessels between the internal mammary arteries and the descending aorta. The presence of neurofibromas or other vascular lesions can also result in rib notching.

The ribs are thin and osteopenic in patients with neuromuscular diseases and osteogenesis imperfecta. Neurofibromatosis patients can have wavy, irregular ribs as part of the skeletal dysplasia present in this disorder.

MEDIASTINUM

The mediastinal structures should be assessed. The thymus is somewhat smaller in the older child in relation to the chest cavity and is not seen so clearly after about 5 years of age. The normal thymus appears prominent between birth and 2 years of age (Fig. 22–7).

Since the trachea is better seen in the older child, the side of the aortic arch is easier to assess than in the neonate. Usually, the trachea deviates away from the side of the aortic arch and the pedicles are denser on the side of the descending thoracic aorta. The descending aorta should not have a convex to the left margin in the normal child. If the aorta does have this configuration, coarctation of the aorta must be considered with

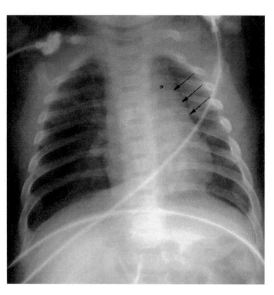

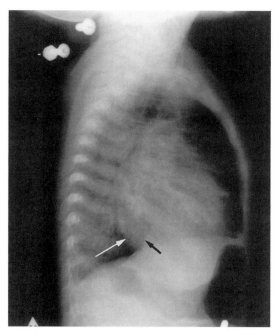

Figure 22–7. Thymus is still border forming in this infant and can be identified by its wavy margin *(arrows)*.

Figure 22–8. Lateral view in this patient with a large left ventricle due to a large left-to-right shunt. Note how the cardiac silhouette intersects the hemidiaphragm *(white arrow)* posterior to the inferior vena cava shadow *(black arrow)*.

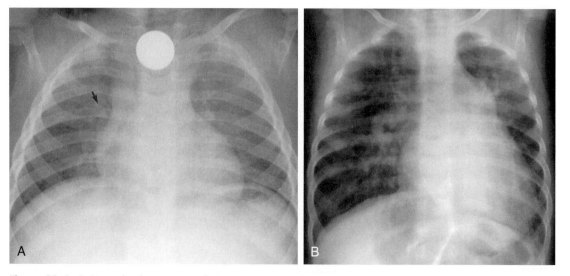

Figure 22–9. A, Normal pulmonary vascularity in a patient with an esophageal coin. The vessel and bronchus are the same size *(arrow)*, and there are no vessels seen below the hemidiaphragms or in the outer one third of the lungs. **B,** Increased pulmonary vascularity in this patient with a left-to-right shunt.

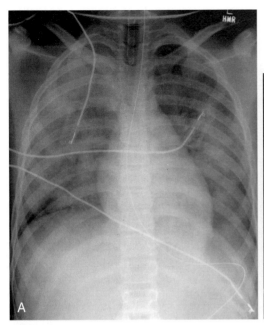 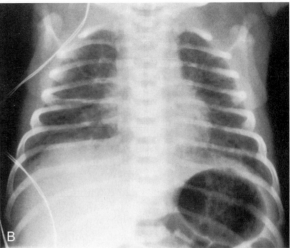

Figure 22–10. A, Fluffy opacity (alveolar filling) in this patient with neurogenic pulmonary edema. **B,** Linear opacity (interstitial prominence) in this neonate with transient tachypnea of the newborn.

the convexity representing poststenotic dilatation of the descending aorta (Fig. 22–6).

Lastly, the cardiac silhouette should be observed for enlargement. The cardiothoracic ratio is the greatest transverse dimension of the heart compared with the transverse dimension of the chest at the inner aspect of the eight ribs. In the older infant and child the cardiothoracic ratio is usually less than 55 percent. On the lateral view the retrosternal area is usually not as filled in as in the infant and toddler, since the thymus is relatively smaller. As a result, right ventricular enlargement can be assessed in older children (Fig. 22–1). Normally the cardiac silhouette fills in the lower one third of the retrosternal air space. Should this space be more than one third filled, it might be due to right ventricular hypertrophy. Left-sided chamber enlargement can be identified on the lateral view by the point where the cardiac silhouette intersects the hemidiaphragm (Fig. 22–8). This point should be anterior to the point where the inferior vena cava intersects the hemidiaphragm. In addition, a line drawn from the anterior tracheal wall straight down to the hemidiaphragm should not intersect the heart.

LUNG PARENCHYMA

Finally, assessment of the lungs should be completed. This evaluation should include both lung opacities and pulmonary vessels. Pulmonary vascularity is normal when a bronchovascular bundle is seen on end and the transverse dimension of the bronchus is the same or larger than the transverse dimension of the adjacent vessel (Fig. 22–9A). In addition, the pulmonary vessels are not prominent in the outer third of the lung or in the lung bases (Fig. 22–9B). Differentiation of pulmonary veins and arteries is difficult depending on how young the child. If possible, the veins can be traced back to the left atrium. If the vessel margins are indistinct, then some degree of pulmonary venous hypertension is usually present.

Lung opacities are usually divided into air space densities (alveolar filling processes) and interstitial densities. In general the air space densities are fluffy opacities (Fig. 22–10A) and the interstitial densities are more linear (Fig. 22–10B). Frequently the pulmonary processes are mixed.

Chapter 23

Respiratory Distress in the Older Infant and Child

Just as in the neonate, there are medical and surgical causes of respiratory distress in the older infant and child. Medical causes are those that require supportive therapy such as antibiotics, bronchodilators, chest physiotherapy, and sometimes artificial ventilation, among others. Commonly encountered causes include the following entities: infections, reactive airways disease, cystic fibrosis, aspiration pneumonia, immune deficiency syndromes, and although rare, pulmonary emboli or other vascular diseases. Surgical causes are those that require surgical intervention such as bronchoscopy or thoracotomy to obtain a cure. Included in this category are intrinsic tracheal pathology, foreign body aspiration, trauma, and masses.

MEDICAL CAUSES OF RESPIRATORY DISTRESS

Infections

Infectious causes can be divided into upper respiratory tract and lower respiratory tract pathology. Causes of upper involvement are mainly epiglottitis, croup, and bacterial tracheitis.

Epiglottitis, which historically has been due to *Haemophilus influenzae*, has almost been eliminated with the advent of the *H. influenzae* type b vaccination. Croup frequently has a viral cause, such as parainfluenza. Bacterial tracheitis can be due to a number of infectious agents including *Streptococcus* and nontypeable *H. influenzae*.

Lower respiratory tract infectious agents in the pediatric population are age-related. During the neonatal period the most common etiologic agent for lower respiratory tract infection is bacterial in origin. The most common etiologic agent from approximately 1 month to 3 months of age includes viral as well as pertussis and *Chlamydia* infections. After 3 months until approximately school age, viral agents are by far the most common infectious agents. Respiratory syncytial virus is most serious in infants under 1 year of age. Other viral agents such as adenovirus and parainfluenza are also important. If bacterial agents are implicated, *H. influenzae* and pneumococcal infections are the most likely. Although *Mycoplasma* is seen in this younger age group, school-age children are more likely to have *Mycoplasma* infections. Viral agents play less of a role in these older children.

Radiographic Patterns of Upper Tract Infection. A frontal and lateral view of the neck is the best way to evaluate the airway in a young infant and child radiographically. The normal anatomy must be known before pathology can be diagnosed (Fig. 23–1). Air must be in the hypopharynx and trachea in order to make full evaluation of the lateral neck. The air serves as a contrast medium against the soft-tissue structures. If there is no air in these structures, as occurs with swallowing, a mass is simulated (Fig. 23–2). On the frontal view, the vocal cords are at approximately the level of the piriform sinuses. Below this level of the cords is the subglottic trachea. The appearance of the subglottic airway has been compared to "square shoulders" (Fig. 23–3).

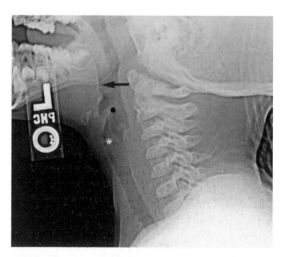

Figure 23–1. Normal view of lateral neck. The epiglottis *(dot)* is at the level of the hyoid bone. The laryngeal ventricle *(asterisk)* separates the false (above) from the true cords (below). Base of tongue *(arrow)* is also seen.

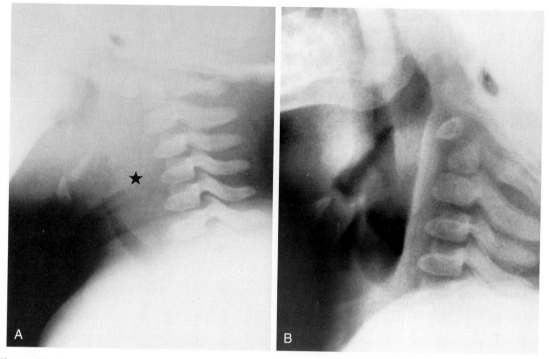

Figure 23–2. A, No air in hypopharynx secondary to swallowing simulates mass *(star).* **B,** Same patient minutes later with air in the hypopharynx and no evidence of mass.

The epiglottis is easily located just posterior to the hyoid bone in the lateral view. It should appear no larger than the lateral of a person's little finger. The folds extending down from the epiglottis, the aryepiglottic folds, should be

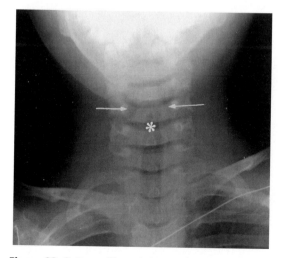

Figure 23–3. Normal frontal view of the airway. The pyriform sinuses *(arrows)* are at the level of the vocal cords. Below this is the subglottic trachea *(asterisk).*

pencil-thin. When epiglotittis is present, the epiglottis and aryepiglottic folds are thickened such that the epiglottis looks like a "thumb" (Fig. 23–4). (Note: Usually films are not obtained in patients who may have epiglottitis because the airway may become completely obstructed during the performance of the radiograph.) If films are necessary, only a lateral view with the patient upright should be obtained.

Croup is best diagnosed on a frontal view. The normal shoulder appearance to the subglottic airway is edematous with croup and assumes the appearance of a "steeple" (Fig. 23–5). The lateral view shows decreased lucency in the subglottic airway. This appearance is not specific for croup but can be seen at times during the normal respiratory cycle and in patients who are recently extubated. Beware of the 30 percent of epiglottitis cases that also have subglottic edema as part of the process. The subglottic edema should be symmetric in croup. If it is not, then a mass should be suspected such as hemangioma or neurofibroma.

Membranous croup is frequently only a bronchoscopic diagnosis. Occasionally, soft-tissue densities that are characteristic of this disorder are seen in the trachea on the lateral view.

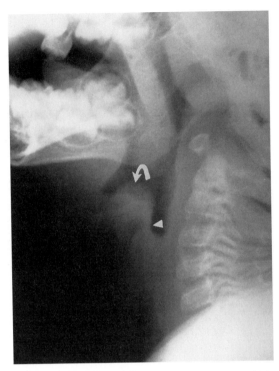

Figure 23–4. Lateral view showing epiglottitis with thickening of both the epiglottis *(curved arrow)* and the aryepiglottic folds *(arrowhead)*.

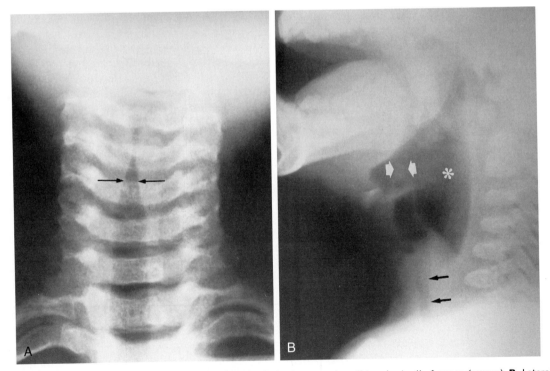

Figure 23–5. A, Frontal view showing the symmetric subglottic narrowing, "steeple sign" of croup *(arrows)*. **B,** Lateral view showing decreased lucency of the subglottic airway *(black arrows)* and ballooning of the hypopharynx *(asterisk)* due to the airway obstruction. The epiglottis is normal *(white arrows)*.

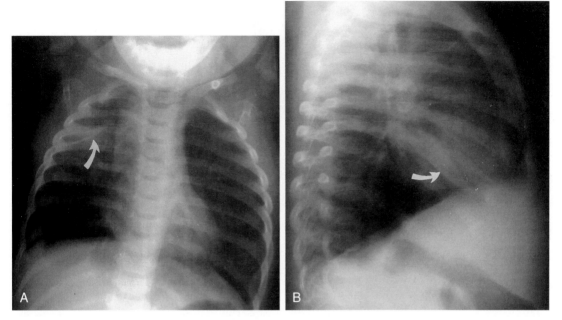

Figure 23–6. A, Typical appearance of patient with viral lower respiratory tract infection causing hyperinflation and linear streaky densities secondary to atelectasis *(arrow)*. **B,** Lateral view confirms hyperinflation and streaky atelectasis *(arrow)*.

Radiographic Patterns of Lower Respiratory Tract Infections. Hyperinflation characterizes the radiographic pattern of viral lower respiratory tract infections (Fig. 23–6). In the young child, hyperinflation is diagnosed by seeing the hemidiaphragm to at least nine posterior ribs of inflation on the frontal view and flattened hemidiaphragms on the lateral. The hyperinflation results from the normal airways in young children being somewhat hypercollapsible on exhalation. When some-

thing compromises the lumens of the airways, such as inflammation or edema as can be seen with viral infections, the airways collapse more than usual on exhalation. Air can get in on inspiration but can't get out on exhalation, which results in air trapping. Air trapping is not specific for viral lower respiratory tract infections but may help in diagnosing the presence of some abnormality in the pulmonary parenchyma. In older children, rib counting no longer works for hy-

Figure 23–7. Bronchiolitis resulting in right upper lobe collapse as demonstrated by the elevated minor fissure *(arrows)*.

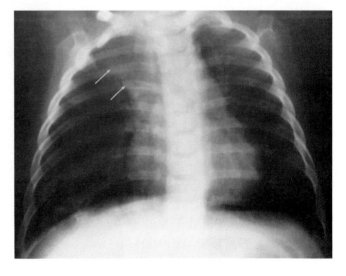

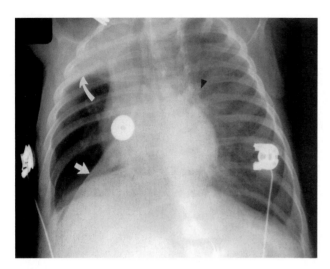

Figure 23–8. Right upper lobe atelectasis is shown with the elevated minor fissure *(curved arrow)* and lower lobe collapse is seen by the major fissure being pulled down and medially *(straight arrow)*. Bronchial wall thickening is also demonstrated *(black arrowhead)*.

perinflation. Instead, flattening of the hemidiaphragms and subjective increased thoracic volumes are used.

Other findings associated with viral agents are areas of atelectasis secondary to mucous plugging and bronchial wall thickening caused by inflammation. Atelectasis is frequently linear in appearance, can cause movement of fissures if extensive enough, and changes rapidly over a matter of hours. When there is right upper lobe collapse, the minor fissure is classically elevated (Fig. 23–7). When there is atelectasis involving an entire lower lobe, the respective major fissure is pulled down and medially (Fig. 23–8) so that it is visible on the frontal radiograph when normally this fissure is only seen on the lateral view. Left upper lobe collapse causes obscuration of the left cardiomediastinal contour. Bronchial wall thickening is best seen when a bronchus is seen in cross section and has the appearance of a donut. The bronchial walls are not normally seen in young children.

The radiographic findings described above are also seen with *Chlamydia* and pertussis and sometimes *Mycoplasma*. Therefore, the age of the patient is extremely important in trying to ascertain the infectious agent causing the lower respiratory tract infection.

With other bacterial agents the appearance is

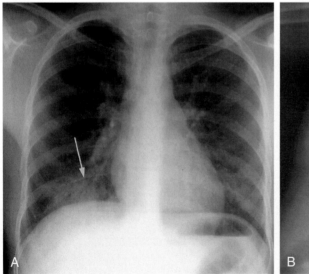

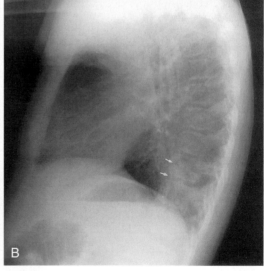

Figure 23–9. A, Right lower lobe bacterial pneumonia in an older child *(arrow)*. No diffuse air trapping is present. **B,** Lateral view shows increased opacity over lower thoracic spine indicative of a lower lobe process *(arrows)*.

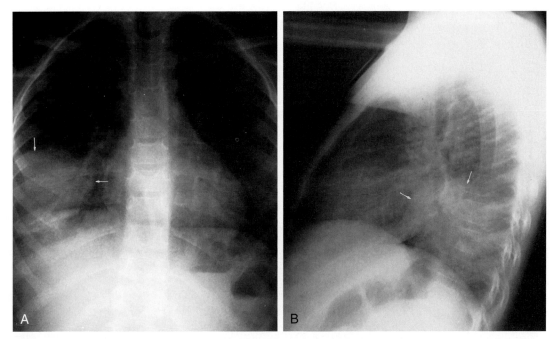

Figure 23–10. A, Typical round pneumonia seen in the right lower lobe *(arrows)*. The margins are slightly irregular. **B,** Opacity over the lower thoracic spine *(arrows)*.

frequently different from that seen with viral processes. There is frequently a focal air space process present, usually without generalized air trapping (Fig. 23–9). The air space process does not change rapidly, as can be seen with atelectasis. Although pleural effusion can be seen in a small percentage of cases due to viral agents, it is more commonly seen in bacterial processes.

A specific appearance of bacterial pneumonia due to pneumococcal infection is that of the "round pneumonia" (Fig. 23–10). This air space process has a rounded appearance with slightly irregular margins and is located primarily in the basilar segments of an upright child or in the dependent segments of a supine infant (i.e., superior segments of the lower lobes). This typically occurs in patients under age 8.

Patients may have respiratory symptoms due to airway compromise incurred by granulomatous disease such as tuberculosis. (Remember: Unilateral hilar adenopathy is indicative of tuberculosis until proven otherwise [Fig. 23–11].)

Reactive Airways Disease

Asthma or reactive airways disease (RAD) is defined as the episodic and reversible broncho-constriction that occurs secondary to hypersensitivity to a variety of stimuli. The radiographic appearance of an acute episode of RAD is indistin-guishable from that seen with viral lower respiratory tract infection. There is generalized air trapping (hyperinflation), bronchial wall thickening, and focal areas of air space density that most often are due to atelectasis. Sometimes air leak phenomena, pneumomediastinum, or pneumothorax develop because of severe bronchospasms (Fig. 23–12).

Since patients with RAD can have superimposed infectious agents, it can be impossible to tell whether the air space process represents atelectasis or bacterial pneumonia. Since atelectasis changes rapidly with time, a repeat radiograph following bronchodilator therapy and chest physiotherapy frequently shows a change in the air space opacities. This indicates atelectasis, which is extremely common in patients with RAD. With more chronic RAD, the bony thorax can assume a barrel shape with an increase in the transverse diameter of the chest as well as an increase in the anteroposterior diameter of the chest on the lateral view. Bronchial wall thickening and patchy areas of atelectasis are still present as in the patients with recent onset of RAD.

Cystic Fibrosis

Cystic fibrosis or mucoviscidosis is an autosomal recessive disease. It affects multiple organ systems because of mucus plugging. This plug-

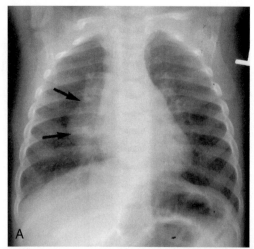

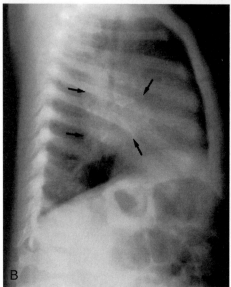

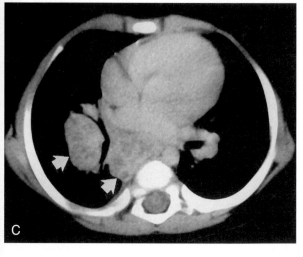

Figure 23–11. A, Frontal view of patient with unilateral hilar adenopathy *(arrows)* secondary to tuberculosis. **B,** Lateral view confirming the presence of the hilar nodes *(arrows).* **C,** CT scan with intravenous enhancement showing both the right hilar and mediastinal nodal mass *(arrows).*

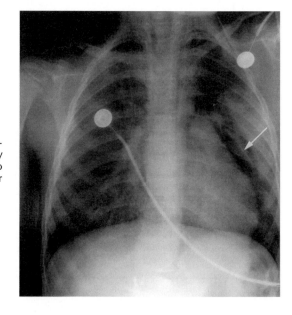

Figure 23–12. Asthmatic patient who had so much bronchospasm that pneumomediastinum occurred as shown by air outlining the thymus *(arrow).* Air space density is also seen in the left midlung that could be either atelectasis or bacterial pneumonia.

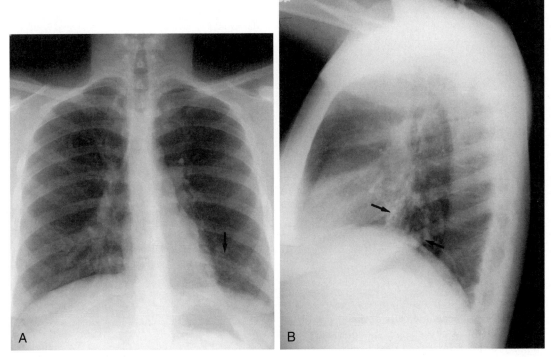

Figure 23–13. Patient with mild pulmonary changes of cystic fibrosis that are indistinguishable from those of viral or reactive airway disease. **A,** Frontal view shows bronchial wall thickening and prominent patchy densities at the left lung base *(arrow)*. **B,** Lateral view confirms the frontal findings of lower lobe abnormality *(arrows)*.

ging is due to a dysfunction of the exocrine glands that causes abnormal secretions. Early in the disease the radiographic appearance is indistinguishable from that seen in viral lower respiratory tract infection and RAD (Fig. 23–13). There is generalized air trapping and bronchial wall thickening as well as atelectasis from mucus plugs. Later there are dilated bronchi (bronchiectasis) filled with mucus plugs and usually marked air trapping that makes the bony thorax barrel shaped (Fig. 23–14). The bronchiectasis tends to be generalized but may be worse in the upper lobes. Late in the disease, pulmonary arterial hypertension is present, which can be identified by enlarged central pulmonary arteries and an enlarged right ventricle as seen on the lateral view. The enlarged right ventricle can be identified by the filling in of the retrosternal clear space by more than the usual one third as seen in the normal child.

Aspiration Pneumonia

Aspiration pneumonia causes radiographic abnormality depending on the position of the patient at the time of the aspiration, as well as on the amount and type of material aspirated. In the

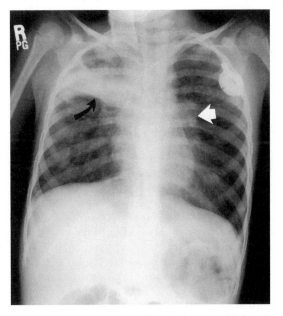

Figure 23–14. Severe cystic fibrosis changes with barrel-shaped chest due to chronic air trapping, chronic right upper lobe collapse *(curved arrow)*, and diffuse bronchial wall thickening with prominent pulmonary arteries *(arrow for left pulmonary artery)* due to pulmonary arterial hypertension.

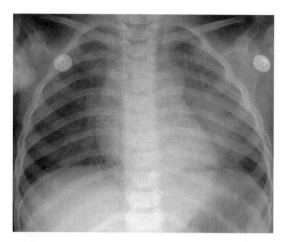

Figure 23–15. Fluffy opacities seen most prominently at the left lung base are a result of acute hydrocarbon aspiration.

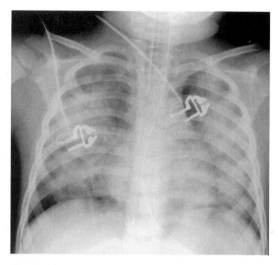

Figure 23–16. Noncardiac pulmonary edema pattern seen in this near drowning patient.

infant who is being fed, usually in the caretaker's left arm, or in the neurologically devastated child who is supine most of the time, the most dependent portion of the thorax is the posterior segment of the right upper lobe. In the upright child, aspiration occurs in the lung bases. Acute aspiration causes air-space processes in the locations described earlier. Chronic aspiration can cause an appearance similar to that of a viral lower respiratory tract infection with bronchial wall thickening and sometimes even bronchiectasis. Three specific types of acute aspiration pneumonia will be described: hydrocarbon aspiration, near drowning, and smoke inhalation.

Hydrocarbon Aspiration. The location of the hydrocarbon aspiration (i.e., kerosene or gasoline) is usually basilar because those children who obtain these substances are usually ambulatory. The hydrocarbons cause a chemical pneumonitis that has the appearance of fluffy opacities acutely (Fig. 23–15) and with time may cavitate into pneumatoceles. The appearance of the opacities may not be visualized for up to 6 hours after the event. The radiographic findings may be present for several days after the patient is clinically well. The patient must also be monitored for superimposed bacterial infection.

Near Drowning. The radiographic appearance is usually that of perihilar air space opacities (Fig. 23–16) with a normal-sized cardiac silhouette (noncardiac pulmonary edema). The radiographic appearance is related to the amount of water aspirated, not to whether it is fresh or salt water.

The severity of the radiographic changes does not necessarily correlate with the patient outcome.

Smoke Inhalation. The radiographic changes, when present, consist of air-space processes as a result of pulmonary edema and hemorrhage. The radiographs may be normal if the inhalation is mild.

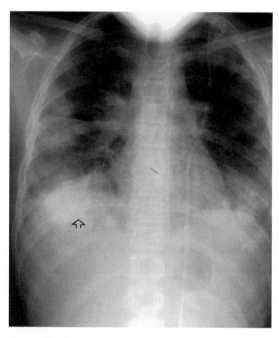

Figure 23–17. Septic pulmonary emboli in this immunocompromised patient with multiple nodules. A few have cavitation consistent with septic emboli *(arrow).*

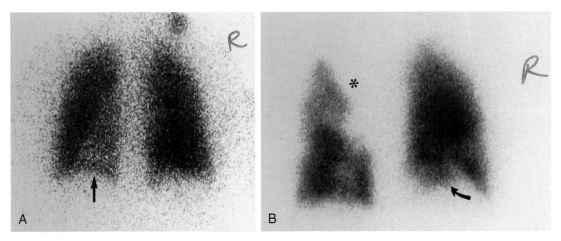

Figure 23–18. Ventilation/perfusion scan—mismatched defect. **A,** Ventilation scan in the posterior projection showing normal ventilation. There is slightly less ventilation where the heart is located *(arrow)*. **B,** Perfusion scan in the posterior projection showing a large perfusion defect in the left upper lobe *(asterisk)* and a smaller defect in the right lower lobe *(curved arrow)*.

Immune Deficiency Syndromes

Immune deficiency syndromes, such as immunoglobulin deficiencies, can cause radiographic findings similar to those discussed under Radiographic Patterns of Lower Respiratory Tract Infections (i.e., bronchial wall thickening and hyperinflation). Air space opacities can be present depending on whether or not an acute superinfection is present.

Pulmonary Emboli

Occasionally pulmonary emboli (PE) cause respiratory distress in the pediatric population. The most common cause is infection due to indwelling catheters such as those seen in immunocompromised patients. Septic PE can be from septic thrombophlebitis. Thrombophlebitis, however, is rare in the pediatric population. Radiographically, plain chest film shows cavitated modules (Fig. 23–17). Other causes of PE can be from tumor thrombus such as that seen with Wilms tumor, which rarely invades the inferior vena cava and embolizes to the lungs. Although rare, noninfected PE can also occur in children. A nuclear medicine ventilation/perfusion ($\dot{V}/\dot{Q}$) scan is the best imaging modality for evaluating the presence or absence of PE. The plain chest radiograph needs to be nearly normal in order for adequate interpretation of the $\dot{V}/\dot{Q}$ scan. For a positive scan there must be a significant ventilation/perfusion mismatch, that is, normal ventilation but abnormal perfusion (Fig. 23–18).

SURGICAL CAUSES OF RESPIRATORY DISTRESS

Tracheal Stenosis and Other Tracheal Pathology

Tracheal stenosis is most frequently seen in the young infant or child who has been intubated for a long time. A typical history is that the infant was born prematurely and required prolonged mechanical ventilation. The stenosis is usually seen in the subglottic airway. Another cause of tracheal narrowing results from granulation tissue that forms during repeated suctioning while the patient is being ventilated. Granulation tissue is usually suspected when persistent atelectasis is seen in babies being mechanically ventilated. The diagnosis is made bronchoscopically.

Other tracheal pathology includes masses in the airway such as papillomas, hemangiomas, and neurofibromas. Extratracheal pathology such as thyroid masses (Fig. 23–19), cystic hygromas (lymphangiomas), or retropharyngeal abscesses can cause such tracheal embarrassment that the patient is in severe respiratory distress.

Retropharyngeal abscesses usually occur in patients who have had either trauma by a penetrating object or have had recent upper respiratory tract infection. These abscesses are diagnosed by seeing prevertebral soft-tissue swelling with airway encroachment in the extended lateral neck (Fig. 23–20). Neck flexion and swallowing causes artifactual soft-tissue swelling (Fig. 23–2A). The diagnosis of abscess is only

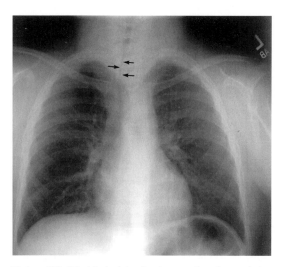

Figure 23–19. Marked tracheal narrowing *(arrows)* due to thyroid carcinoma.

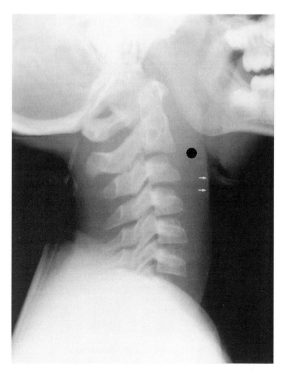

Figure 23–20. Retropharyngeal swelling. On a fully extended neck, the prevertebral soft tissues *(dot)* are too wide (greater than the AP diameter of C2). There is mass effect on the airway *(arrows)*. This swelling turned out to be abscess formation.

made when air is seen in the prevertebral soft tissues on plain film or as an enhancing mass on a CT of the neck.

Vascular rings also cause airway embarrassment. Virtually all symptomatic vascular rings are seen in patients with right aortic arches. There are two types, double aortic arch and right arch with an aberrant left subclavian where the ductus ligament forms the ring. The diagnosis of vascular

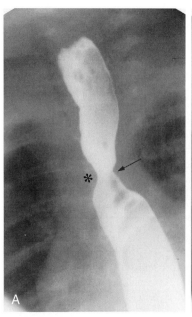

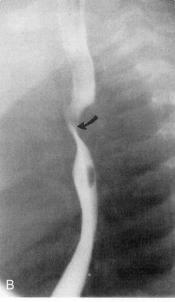

Figure 23–21. Vascular ring. **A,** Frontal view of barium esophagram with mass effect on both sides of the esophagus from vascular impressions of the right aortic arch *(asterisk)* and ductus ligament *(arrow)*. **B,** Lateral view showing posterior impression on esophagus due to the aberrant origin of the left subclavian artery *(arrow)*.

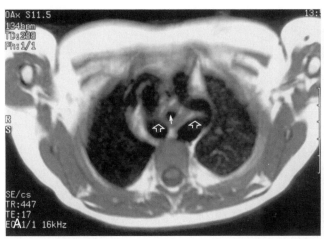
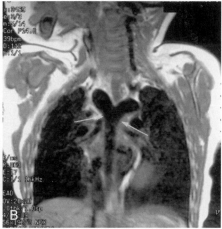

Figure 23–22. Vascular ring. **A,** Axial T1 view where fat is white shows the double arch *(open arrows)* encircling the airway *(solid arrow).* **B,** Coronal T1 view where the double arches join to form the descending aorta *(arrows).*

ring is usually suspected on a barium esophagram. All patients will have identical vascular impressions on the esophagus regardless of the type of vascular ring (Fig. 23–21). MRI of the chest is the best imaging modality for distinguishing types of vascular rings (Fig. 23–22).

Chronic esophageal foreign bodies can result in mass effect on the trachea and result in airway symptoms due to the inflammatory reaction caused in the esophagus (Fig. 23–23). It is un-

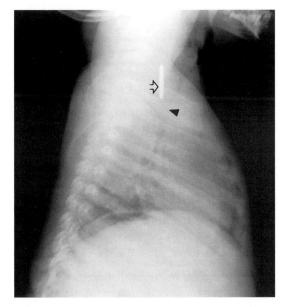

Figure 23–23. Esophageal foreign body, a coin *(open arrow)*, which has caused inflammation and resultant mass effect and narrowing *(arrowhead)* of the trachea.

usual for the patient to have esophageal symptoms from a chronic esophageal foreign body. As a general rule, all patients with new onset respiratory symptoms should have a chest radiograph to exclude foreign body ingestion.

Foreign Body Aspiration

Foreign body aspiration is typically seen in young infants who are in the "vacuum cleaner phase." This is where all objects on the floor are scooped up and put into the mouth. Peak age range for this behavior is 1 to 2 years.

Aspirated foreign bodies are rarely opaque (Fig. 23–24). Therefore indirect signs of a foreign body in the airway must be sought. Foreign body aspiration acutely causes air trapping focally (i.e., one lung, one lobe, or one segment). Either lung can be affected. The mechanism of air trapping is similar to that seen with viral lower respiratory tract infections in that the airways collapse slightly with normal exhalation. With a foreign body that does not completely occlude the airway, air can get in around the object but air cannot get out, resulting in air trapping. Atelectasis results when the foreign body has been in the airway for several days and edema has occluded it. Sometimes a postobstructive pneumonia is associated. Although the most common cause of atelectasis is mucus plugging, any persistent atelectasis should raise concern of an aspirated foreign body. Likewise, an air-space process that was thought to represent pneumonia but that also demonstrates evidence of volume loss (atelectasis) could be indicative of an aspirated foreign body. However,

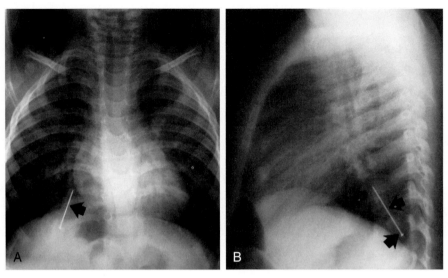

Figure 23–24. Aspirated radiopaque foreign body. **A,** Frontal view of right lower lobe aspirated foreign body, a straight-pin *(arrow)*. **B,** Lateral view confirming the location of the opaque foreign body *(arrows)*.

it is most likely mucus plugging that is causing the atelectasis.

Radiographically, focal air trapping should be sought. That portion of the lung that is air trapping should be more lucent than the rest of the lung for two reasons. One, there is more air, and two, there is physiologic shunting of pulmonary blood flow away from the obstructed piece of lung (Fig. 23–25). Sometimes the air trapping is not readily obvious on the plain frontal view. In these cases, exhalation views are necessary. An obstructed portion of lung does not vary with inhalation or exhalation. In the cooperative child, an exhalation view can be obtained and compared with the inhalation view. In the uncooperative child, decubitus views are best for demostrating air trapping. The decubitus views work by having the side down exhale and the side up inhale (Fig. 23–26). Both decubitus views are obtained and then compared to assess for exhalation on both sides. Even if the views obtained show no evidence of focal air trapping, the patient should still undergo bronchoscopy if clinical suspicion is high.

Trauma

Trauma results in entities such as lung contusions, traumatic pulmonary pseudocysts, rib fractures, and although rare, traumatic diaphragmatic hernias. Lung contusions are frequently seen in younger children who also have abdominal trauma. When they are present, morbidity, and mortality are increased. Radiographically, lung contusions appear as air-space opacities that usually become larger and denser within 24 to 48 hours after injury (Fig. 23–27). Contusions can cavitate.

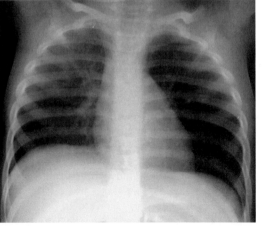

Figure 23–25. Acutely aspirated nonopaque foreign body caused increased lucency to the left lung due to the obstruction of the left main stem bronchus.

Traumatic pulmonary pseudocysts are actual lacerations in the lung that occur at the time of injury and result in a cyst that appears immediately (Fig. 23–28). With time the pseudocysts resolve spontaneously. The pathophysiology behind the pseudocysts is that the bony thorax has intrinsic elasticity in the young child. At the time

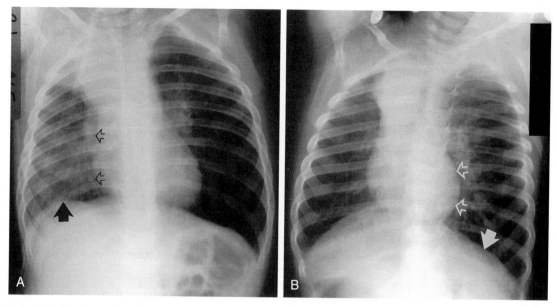

Figure 23–26. Acute airway foreign body aspiration on left. **A,** Right-side-down decubitus view shows that the hemidi-aphragm on the right moves up *(solid arrow)* and the mediastinum falls slightly toward the right *(open arrows)*. **B,** Left-side-down decubitus shows that the left hemidiaphragm stays down *(solid arrow)* and the mediastinum does not fall to the left *(open arrows)*, resulting in air trapping.

of the injury, the thorax springs back into shape. This frequently occurs without bony injury, but the lung itself can tear. Traumatic pulmonary pseudocysts are characteristically seen in patients under the age of 8.

Rib fractures are not nearly as common as a result of trauma in the young child as in adolescents and adults. The thorax deforms with injury but springs back to its original shape without much actual fracturing. Therefore, when a young child is seen with several rib fractures, nonaccidental trauma should be considered. The most important complication of rib fracture is pneumo-

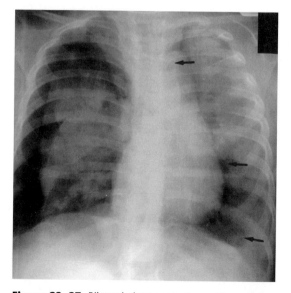

Figure 23–27. Bilateral chest contusions with pneumo-thoraces, right much greater than left. The relative area of lucency *(arrows)* adjacent to the left heart border is the anteromedial pneumothorax. The right is much larger.

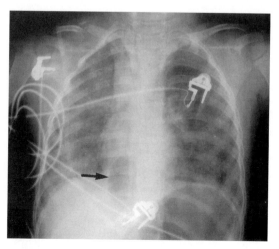

Figure 23–28. Traumatic pulmonary pseudocyst *(arrow)* caused by a tear in the lung. Note the fractured right clavicle. No rib fractures can be seen.

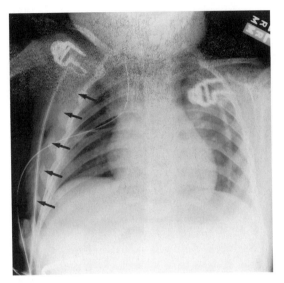

Figure 23–29. An unusually young child that suffered several rib fractures *(arrows)* and resultant pneumothorax that was treated by chest tube.

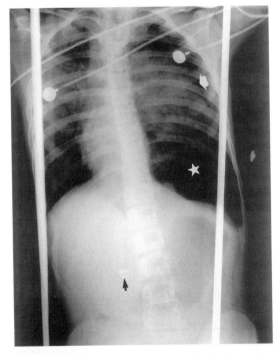

Figure 23–30. Trauma patient with left-sided pneumothorax with a large basilar component *(star)* due to the supine position of the patient. The pneumothorax is so large that it can be seen laterally *(white arrow)* as well. Note the tooth in the abdomen *(black arrow)* that was knocked out and swallowed.

thorax (Fig. 23–29). In a supine patient, regardless of age, pneumothorax collects anteromedially and basilarly in the chest (Fig. 23–30). However, in the upright patient the pneumothorax is seen over the lung apex.

Posttraumatic diaphragmatic hernias are more commonly located on the left side, as are the congenital variety. They are suspected on the basis of the plain chest radiograph that shows an abnormally elevated contour of the hemidiaphragm. The stomach is the most frequently herniated organ. Unenhanced MRI can aid in the diagnosis, if necessary, because of the ability to image in the coronal plane, which can show diaphramatic discontinuity.

Masses or Mass Effects

Masses in the chest can cause respiratory distress. Most masses are located in the mediastinum. Lung parenchymal masses are most commonly due to metastases. Rarely, lung abscesses (Fig. 23–31) and intrapulmonary bronchogenic cysts are present and can cause respiratory distress. Other lung masses can cause respiratory distress either due to their sheer size or to superimposed infection. Cystic adenomatoid malformations (CAM) frequently present with recurrent infections (Fig. 23–32) in the older infant and child as opposed to the neonate, where they present

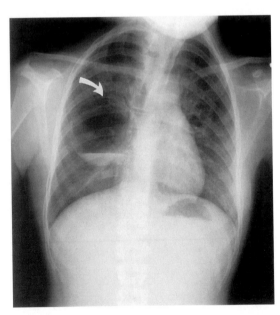

Figure 23–31. Infected cystic area *(arrow)* in the right lung proved to be a lung abscess at surgery.

because of the mass effect of the CAM. Primary tumors of the lung are rare in pediatrics.

Mediastinal masses are diagnosed radiographically by their location as to anterior, middle, or posterior mediastinal. Masses in the mediastinum are well defined with sharp outlines that are convex toward the parenchyma, whereas lung parenchymal processes tend to have an irregular outline.

The compartments of the mediastinum are divided by imaginary lines on the lateral view of the chest as follows:

- From the inferior manubrial notch to the hemidiaphragm (to include the retrosternal clear space) is the anterior mediastinum
- A line parallel and just anterior to the spine defines the posterior mediastinum

- Between these two lines is the middle mediastinum

Localizing the processes, whether mediastinal or parenchymal, on the frontal view takes advantage of the "silhouette sign" where two opacities of the same density, when adjacent to each other, silhouette the interface between them. For example, when the paraspinous line, which is a posterior structure, is silhouetted out, the process is then localized to the posterior part of the chest. If the heart margin is obscured, the process is in the anterior mediastinum. If the aortic arch is obscured, then there is a middle mediastinal process present.

In the anterior mediastinum, the masses are remembered by the mnemonic of the "terrible Ts," which includes teratoma, terrible lymphoma (Fig.

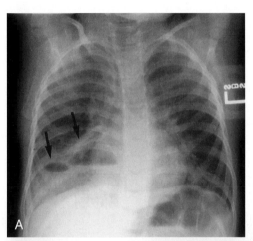

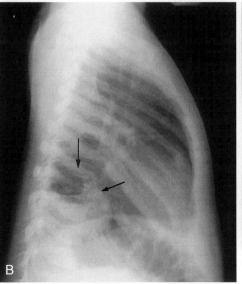

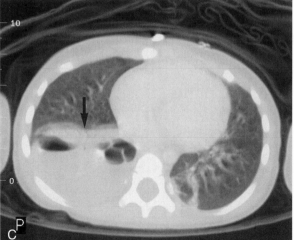

Figure 23–32. A, Infected cystic adenomatoid malformation (CAM) in the right lower lobe with numerous air-fluid levels in it *(arrows).* **B,** Lateral view confirming the location *(arrows).* **C,** Subsequent CT scan showing the extent of the CAM *(arrow).*

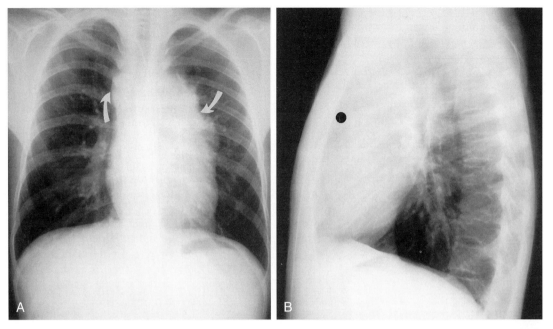

Figure 23–33. Anterior mediastinal mass that was Hodgkin's lymphoma at biopsy. **A,** Lobular mass *(arrows)* that would simulate a thymus in a much younger child. **B,** Filling in of the retrosternal clear space *(dot)* that normally would be filled with air in this older child.

23–33), thymoma or masses involving the thymus, and, although rare, thyroid abnormalities. These masses comprise 30 percent of mediastinal tumors. Anterior mediastinal masses tend to push the trachea, usually posteriorly, and they can also compress the tracheal lumen, which causes respi-

ratory distress. Imaging these patients is best performed with plain chest radiograph and chest CT performed with intravenous contrast. The intravenous contrast material is necessary to sort out mediastinal structures from possible pathology. (A word of warning: Sometimes putting these pa-

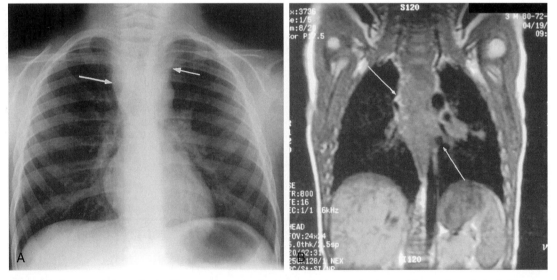

Figure 23–34. A, Subtle mediastinal increased opacity due to lymphadenopathy *(arrows)* from tuberculosis. **B,** The mass of nodes is much better visualized on this T1-weighted coronal MRI scan *(arrows).*

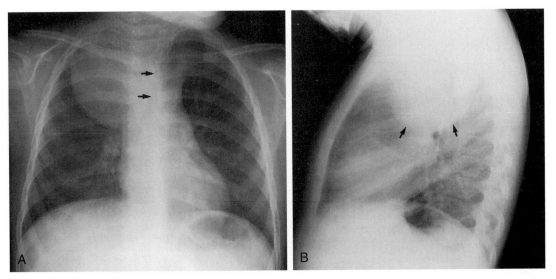

Figure 23–35. A, Bronchogenic cyst so large that it compromised the airway *(arrows)* and had to be resected. Note the sharp borders of this mediastinal mass. **B,** Lateral view shows the huge volume of the mass *(arrows).*

tients in the supine position for the CT scan can aggravate the patient's respiratory distress because of the already compromised airway.)

The middle mediastinum contains masses related to lymphadenopathy (Fig. 23–34), vascular processes such as aneurysms (rare in children), and airway pathology such as bronchogenic cysts and bronchopulmonary foregut malformations. Bronchogenic cysts are the most common masses in this location. They are usually asymptomatic

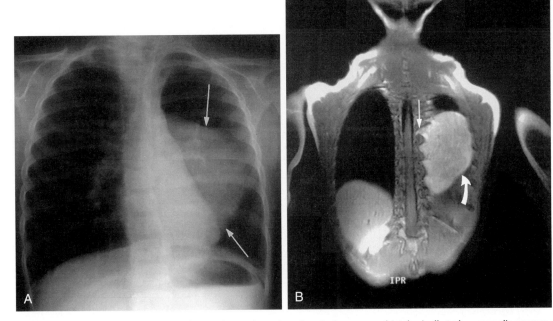

Figure 23–36. A, Posterior mediastinal mass *(arrows)* causing rib splaying proven histologically to be a ganglioneuroma. **B,** T1-weighted MRI sequence demonstrated that the mass *(curved arrow)* extended into the neural foramen *(straight arrow)* but not to the spinal canal.

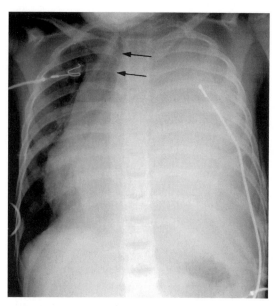

Figure 23–37. Huge malignant pleural effusion resulting in mediastinal shift *(arrows)*.

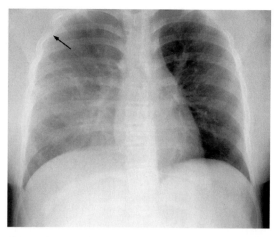

Figure 23–38. Haziness to the right hemithorax is due to pleural effusion layering posteriorly. There is slight displacement of the lung from the inner aspect of the ribs by the effusion *(arrow)*.

and detected on a plain chest radiograph that was taken for other reasons. Occasionally, the cyst lining can secrete mucous that can cause the cyst to grow and cause symptoms by compressing the airway (Fig. 23–35).

Approximately 95 percent of posterior mediastinal masses are neurogenic in origin with neuroblastoma and neurofibromas being the most common. These masses are not clearly seen on the lateral examination but can be localized easily on the frontal view because of silhouetting of the posterior paraspinous line and, on occasion, because of either rib erosion or rib splaying due to tumor growth (Fig. 23–36A). Once diagnosed, other imaging modalities are used besides the chest radiograph including thoracic unenhanced MRI to evaluate for possible spinal canal invasion, which is a complication of many of these neurogenic tumors (Fig. 23–36B). Chest CT can be reserved to evaluate bony abnormality, but it is rarely used in this capacity.

Pleural effusions, when large enough, can cause respiratory compromise due to mediastinal shift and compromise of both the ipsilateral and contralateral lungs. Most large effusions in the child are due to infectious causes. Occasionally, however, the pleural effusions are due to underlying malignancy, usually lymphoma (Fig. 23–37). In the evaluation for pleural effusion, if the whole hemithorax is opaque, ultrasound can confirm the presence of effusion and possible septations if thoracentesis could not be successfully performed. When there is less than complete opacification, bilateral decubitus views can be done. When the involved side is dependent, the amount of free effusion can be estimated. However, when the involved side is not dependent, the degree of loculation can also be determined. (Note: When the pleural effusion is not that large, it can cause hazy increased opacity to the affected hemithorax in the supine patient [Fig. 23–38].)

Chapter 24

The Child with Congenital Heart Disease

DIFFERENTIATING CYANOTIC FROM ACYANOTIC CONGENITAL HEART DISEASE

The approach to the differential of congenital heart disease (CHD) in any child requires categorization. A common way of viewing CHD is by first considering whether the patient is cyanotic or acyanotic. If the child is cyanotic, the pulmonary blood flow must be assessed. If pulmonary blood flow is decreased, then a severe right-sided obstructive lesion such as pulmonary atresia must be present. If pulmonary blood flow is increased in the cyanotic infant, then admixture lesions such as transposition of the great vessels must be considered. The cardiac silhouette is usually enlarged in both conditions. The right heart is large in severe right-sided obstructive lesions (Fig. 24–1), and the whole cardiac silhouette is enlarged in admixture lesions due to the increased blood flow going through it (Fig. 24–2). Most patients with cyanotic congenital heart lesions have already been identified in the neonatal period, although tetralogy of Fallot can present later. Radiographically, in patients with tetralogy of Fallot, the cardiac silhouette is frequently normal with normal to slightly decreased pulmonary blood flow and a concave pulmonary outflow tract (non-border-forming pulmonary outflow tract) with prominent aortic knob.

If the patient is acyanotic, the pulmonary blood flow must again be assessed. If the blood flow is increased, then a left-to-right shunt should be considered, such as ventricular septal defect. The pulmonary outflow tract is also prominent because of the increased blood flow through it. The cardiac silhouette is increased in size as well, also because of the increased amount of blood going through it (Fig. 24–3). If the pulmonary blood flow is normal, a valvular lesion or aortic coarctation must be considered. Initially, the cardiac silhouette is normal size. If the patient's condition has progressed to congestive heart failure, then

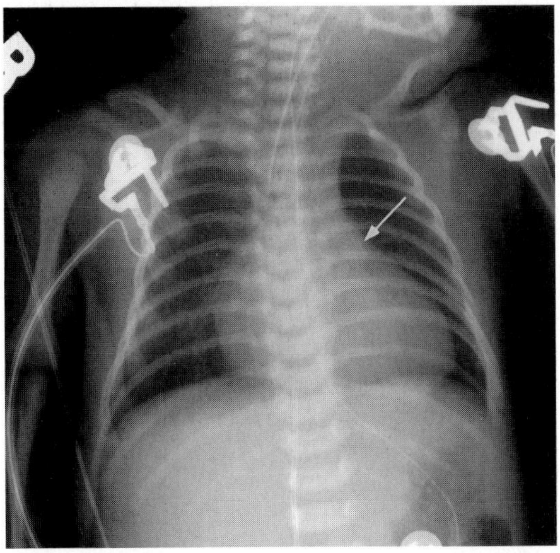

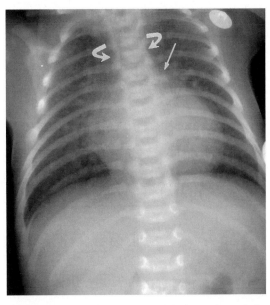

Figure 24–2. Neonate with typical findings of an admixture lesion with increased pulmonary blood flow but a non-border-forming pulmonary outflow tract *(straight arrow)*. There is also stress atrophy of the thymus as seen by the narrow superior mediastinum *(curved arrows)*.

Figure 24–1. Neonate with severe right-sided obstructive lesion resulting in an enlarged cardiac silhouette, concave (non-border-forming) pulmonary outflow tract *(arrow)*, and oligemic lungs (too black).

139

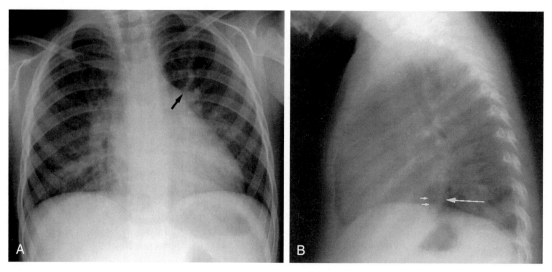

Figure 24–3. A, Patient with left-to-right shunt with enlarged cardiac silhouette, prominent pulmonary blood flow, and convex (border-forming) pulmonary outflow tract *(arrow)*. **B,** Lateral confirms enlarged cardiac silhouette with heart shadow *(large arrow)* projecting posterior to the inferior vena cava shadow *(small arrows)*.

the left-sided obstructive lesions (i.e., aortic stenosis and coarctation) have resulted in left heart failure. (Pulmonary stenosis rarely results in right heart failure.) Other abnormalities such as cardiomyopathies versus a pericardial effusion should also be considered. Radiographically, these patients have enlarged cardiac silhouettes and normal to ill-defined pulmonary vessels (Fig. 24–4).

Out of the neonatal period, most of the patients with congenital heart disease will present with an acyanotic lesion. Therefore, only the acyanotic child will be discussed in this chapter, because those with cyanotic lesions are discussed in Chapter 4.

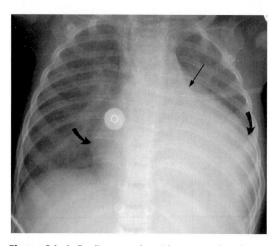

Figure 24–4. Cardiomyopathy with a massively enlarged cardiac silhouette *(curved arrows)* and ill-defined pulmonary vascularity. The cardiac silhouette is so large that it is compressing the left lower lobe bronchus, resulting in left lower lobe collapse *(straight arrow)*.

ACYANOTIC SHUNTS

After the pulmonary vascular resistance drops sufficiently, the uncomplicated acyanotic shunts start to present both clinically and radiographically, that is, shunting of pulmonary blood flow starts going from left to right through congenital defects. The amount of pulmonary blood flow depends on the size of the shunt. The ratio of pulmonary to systemic blood flow determines whether or not the radiographs will be abnormal. This ratio needs to be at least 2:1 in order to see an increase in the pulmonary blood flow radiographically.

All these lesions have a common radiographic appearance in that the pulmonary outflow tract is prominent due to the increased flow through it. The pulmonary outflow tract is border-forming with convexity to the left. Increased pulmonary blood flow can be assessed by comparing the transverse dimension of a vessel with its accompanying bronchus. Normally, these two should be similar in size. In addition, the pulmonary vessels should normally be invisible in the outer third of the lungs and also at the lung bases. Therefore, in patients with acyanotic shunts, the pulmonary vessels should be larger than their accompanying bronchus and they should be visible in the outer portions of the lungs (Fig. 24–3).

The lesions considered in this category are ventricular septal defect (VSD), atrial septal defect (ASD), patent ductus arteriosus (PDA), and endocardial cushion defect (ECD or atrioventricular defect, abbreviated AVC). These lesions are differentiated radiographically on the basis of chamber enlargement.

Ventricular Septal Defects

The ventricular septal defects (VSD) present the earliest because of the high-pressure chambers that are involved. Radiographically, the left atrium and left ventricle are enlarged. Left atrial enlargement is diagnosed by seeing the left main stem bronchus displaced posteriorly by the left atrium (Fig. 24–5). Since a VSD is an intracardiac shunt, the aortic knob is usually not apparent with the pulmonary outflow tract being enlarged. The small defects, not visible on plain chest radiograph, can close spontaneously in the vast majority of the cases. The larger defects are closed surgically, usually before 1 year of age and before the onset of Eisenmenger physiology, that is, right-to-left shunting through the defect because of increased pulmonary vascular resistance that can result from prolonged increased flow to the pulmonary vascular bed in the unrepaired shunt.

Atrial Septal Defects

Atrial septal defects (ASD) usually present later because of the low-pressure chambers involved. ASD is more common in girls. There are several types of atrial septal defects with the most common being the septum secundum. The chest radiograph is frequently normal because the shunts are not that large. If the defect is large enough, the right atrium and right ventricle are enlarged and not the left atrium (Fig. 24–6). Right atrial enlargement is diagnosed by seeing a prominent right heart border. Again, since the defect is an intracardiac one, the aortic knob is usually inconspicuous with a prominent pulmonary outflow tract.

Patent Ductus Arteriosus

Patent ductus arteriosus (PDA) is a persistence of an in utero communication between the pulmonary arteries and the descending thoracic aorta. Most of the time this lesion is asymptomatic and found clinically only on the basis of a continuous murmur. PDA mimics VSD radiographically in that the left-sided chambers are enlarged. However, since PDA is an extracardiac shunt, the aortic knob and the pulmonary outflow tract are enlarged. This distinguishing feature may be hidden behind a prominent thymus. Therefore, if the ra-

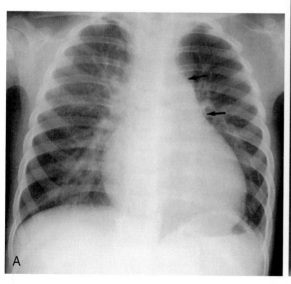
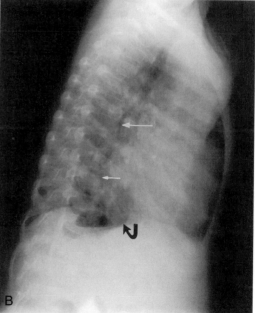

Figure 24–5. Ventricular septal defect. **A,** Enlarged cardiac silhouette, increased pulmonary vascularity, border-forming pulmonary outflow tract *(arrows).* **B,** Enlarged left-sided chambers. Displaced left main stem bronchus *(large arrow)* by left atrium and enlarged left ventricle *(small arrow)* behind inferior vena cava shadow *(curved arrow).*

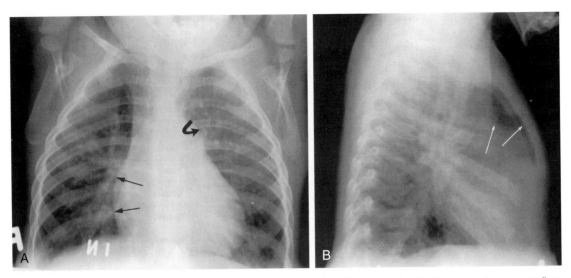

Figure 24–6. Atrial septal defect. **A,** Prominent right atrial shadow *(straight arrows)*, border-forming pulmonary outflow tract *(curved arrow)*, and increased pulmonary vascularity. **B,** Prominent right ventricle, which encroaches on the retrosternal clear space *(arrows)*, but no left-sided chamber enlargement.

diograph has the appearance of a ventricular septal defect, PDA must also be considered.

Endocardial Cushion Defect

The last type of left-to-right shunt is the endocardial cushion defect (ECD), which has a strong association with Down syndrome. Of the congenital heart lesions seen with trisomy 21, nearly half are an ECD. Therefore, in addition to evaluating the chest for the congenital heart lesion, there should

also be an investigation into the radiographic findings seen in Down syndrome such as 11 pairs of ribs, double manubrial ossification center, and bell-shaped thorax. The bell-shaped appearance to the thorax, seen in the neonatal period, becomes somewhat square-shaped later (Fig. 24–7).

Endocardial cushion defects can be partial or complete types. The partial type consists of an ostium primum defect, which is a low type of atrial septal defect, and a cleft mitral valve that is insufficient. Because of the ASD, there is right

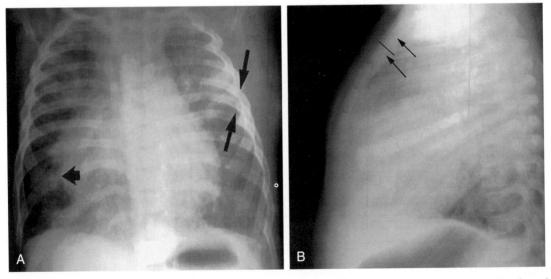

Figure 24–7. Endocardial cushion defect in Down syndrome patient. **A,** The thoracic cage is somewhat square shaped. The right atrium is markedly enlarged *(short arrow)*. Postthoracotomy rib changes *(long arrows)* from previous coarctation repair. **B,** Double manubrial ossification center *(arrows)* in the same patient.

atrial enlargement. In addition, there is left atrial enlargement because of the insufficient mitral valve. Therefore, biatrial enlargement is typical of the partial type of ECD. The pulmonary vascularity is not as great as with the complete type and is similar to that seen with the usual septum secundum type of atrial septal defect.

With the complete type of ECD, there is still the ostium primum ASD with an additional high VSD and a single atrioventricular valve common to the right ventricle and left ventricle. Shunting between the left atrium and right atrium frequently occurs as well as between the left ventricle and right atrium and also between the left ventricle and right ventricle. Therefore, the right-sided chambers are markedly enlarged with a normal-sized left atrium. The pulmonary vascularity is enlarged with a prominent pulmonary outflow tract and a diminutive aortic knob because the ECD is an intracardiac shunt.

ACYANOTIC PATIENT WITH NORMAL PULMONARY BLOOD FLOW WITH OR WITHOUT PULMONARY EDEMA

Included in this category are mainly left-sided obstructive lesions (aortic stenosis, mitral stenosis, and aortic coarctation), cardiomyopathies, and pulmonary stenosis. Pericardial effusion can also cause a similar appearance. Radiographically, this group of lesions has a common appearance in that the cardiac silhouette and pulmonary vascularity are normal at first, and later the cardiac silhouette becomes enlarged. The pulmonary vascularity is indistinct when there is heart failure (Fig. 24–8). The congestive heart failure occurs

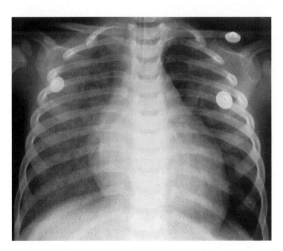

Figure 24–8. Cardiomyopathy with enlarged cardiac silhouette and ill-defined pulmonary vascularity.

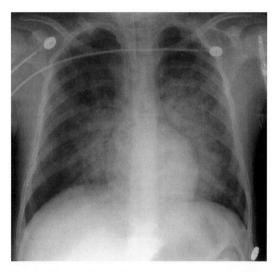

Figure 24–9. Noncardiac pulmonary edema with a normal-sized cardiac silhouette and the diffuse alveolar filling process of pulmonary edema in this severely neurologically damaged teenager.

only with left-sided obstructive lesions and cardiomyopathies but not with pulmonary stenosis. Noncardiac pulmonary edema has a normal-sized cardiac silhouette (Fig. 24–9).

Aortic Stenosis

Aortic stenosis that presents out of the neonatal period and in the older child is usually asymptomatic and is only found because of a murmur. The obstruction to the left ventricle can be at the valvular level, subvalvular level, or supravalvular level. Valvular aortic stenosis is the most common level of obstruction and can be congenital with a bicuspid aortic valve or acquired due to rheumatic valvular disease. Frequently, with the acquired type, there is valvular insufficiency as well. With pure valvular stenosis without insufficiency, the radiographic findings are that of a normal-sized cardiac silhouette with a prominent ascending aorta due to poststenotic dilatation (Fig. 24–10). The poststenotic dilatation results from the eccentric "jet" of blood passing through the stenotic valve, which dilates the supravalvular aorta over time. Therefore, the ascending aorta is seen to the right of the spine, which is abnormal in children. The left ventricle enlarges with left ventricular failure or valvular insufficiency, or both (Fig. 24–11).

Mitral Stenosis

Mitral stenosis (MS) can be congenital or acquired, with the acquired form much more com-

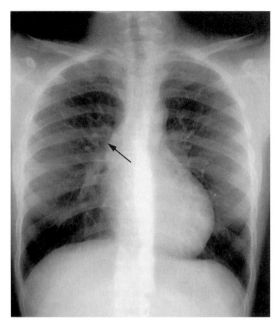

Figure 24–10. Pure aortic stenosis with a normal-sized cardiac silhouette and prominent ascending aorta *(arrow)*.

mon. Acquired MS is usually due to rheumatic heart disease, which can also involve other valves, but the mitral is most common. The radiographic findings are those of left atrial enlargement and pulmonary venous congestion in pure mitral stenosis. With mitral regurgitation, the left ventricle is enlarged as well. Left atrial enlargement causes

posterior displacement of the left main stem bronchus on the lateral view. In adults with left atrial enlargement, the right aspect of the left atrium is seen ("double density" sign), and it is pathologic. However, this finding is usually normal in children. Late in the course of mitral stenosis, the left main stem bronchus is uplifted on the frontal view with splaying of the carina. In addition, there is prominence to the left atrial appendage, which causes a border-forming third bump along the left heart border. The first and second bumps are the aortic arch and the pulmonary outflow tract, respectively. The third bump can be seen in approximately 5 percent of normal people.

Cardiomyopathies

Cardiomyopathies present radiographically similar to the presentation of valvular lesions. Early in the course of the disease, the left ventricle is the first chamber to dilate and fail. The left atrium then dilates because there is usually mitral valve incompetence. This results from mitral annulus dilatation that occurred because of the dilated left ventricle. Then the right-sided chambers dilate, which causes global cardiomegaly in the vast majority of cardiomyopathies (Fig. 24–12). The pulmonary vascularity is normal until the patient goes into congestive heart failure, whereupon the vessels become indistinct.

The most common cause of cardiomyopathy in the older child is viral myocarditis as seen with

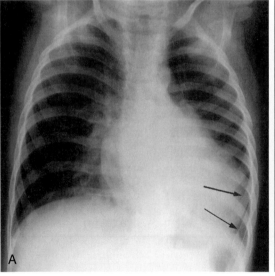

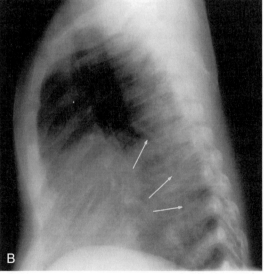

Figure 24–11. A, Marfan syndrome patient with aortic valve insufficiency resulting in a markedly enlarged left ventricle as demonstrated by the "LV" configuration to the heart *(arrows)*. **B,** Lateral view confirming the enlarged left-sided chambers *(arrows)*. The left atrium has become enlarged secondary to mitral annulus dilatation and resultant mitral valve insufficiency.

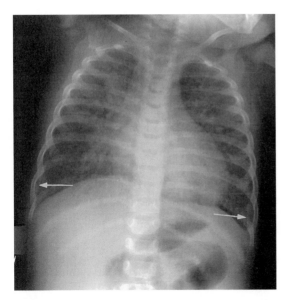

Figure 24–12. Cardiomyopathy with enlarged cardiac silhouette, bilateral pleural effusions *(arrows)*, and pulmonary vascular ill definition.

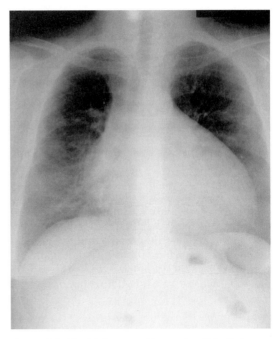

Figure 24–13. Adolescent with a pericardial effusion resulting in an enlarged cardiac silhouette. Diagnosis was confirmed by cardiac echo.

coxsackievirus. Other causes of cardiomyopathy include the following:

- Glycogen storage disease, in which abnormal glycogen accumulation occurs in the endocardium
- Endocardial fibroelastosis, which is a thickening of the endocardium that leads to a noncompliant left ventricle (usually a diagnosis of exclusion in its primary form)
- Kawasaki syndrome, which is a syndrome causing vasculitis throughout the body but especially the coronary arteries
- Aberrant origin of the left coronary artery where the coronary artery arises from the pulmonary artery and blood is shunted from the left coronary artery to the pulmonary system with resultant ischemia and infarction of the left ventricle
- In the adolescent who has had chemotherapy as a young child, specifically adriamycin, cardiomyopathy can result

Pericardial Effusion

Radiographically, pericardial effusion can mimic the lesions discussed earlier by causing a markedly enlarged cardiac silhouette with normal pulmonary blood flow. The appearance of the cardiac silhouette has been compared to a water bottle (Fig. 24–13). Although there have been attempts to diagnose the effusion on plain film by certain radiographic signs, the best way to make the diagnosis of the effusion is with a cardiac echo.

Pulmonary Stenosis

The appearance of pulmonary stenosis depends on the child's age at presentation. Those who present in the neonatal period with critical pulmonic stenosis have an enlarged cardiac silhouette with decreased pulmonary blood flow. Those who present as a child have a normal appearing chest radiograph. Those patients who present in late adolescence and adulthood demonstrate prominence of the pulmonary outflow tract and prominence to the left pulmonary artery. The prominent pulmonary outflow tract is due to poststenotic dilatation that occurs because of the eccentric jet of blood flow through the valve. (Warning: A prominent pulmonary outflow tract can be seen normally in adolescent females.) The "jet" also results in prominence of the left pulmonary artery, as well. The remainder of the more peripheral pulmonary blood flow is normal. The right ventricle in these patients is enlarged, as demonstrated on the lateral view with the cardiac silhouette taking up more space than usual in the retrosternal clear space.

Chapter 25

The Child or Adolescent with Abdominal Pain

Abdominal pain is divided into medical and surgical causes. In general, the conditions discussed will be imaged first with plain radiographs. Usually these consist of a supine abdominal film, an upright or decubitus view to detect air-fluid levels and free air and a chest radiograph to also observe for free air and any pneumonic process that might cause referred pain into the abdomen. As in the chest, a system needs to be in place in order to evaluate the plain radiograph of the abdomen.

EVALUATING ABDOMINAL PAIN

Bowel Gas Pattern

In the neonate, the small and large bowels are indistinguishable. Once the infant becomes up-right, the small bowel gas passes through and the colon becomes more recognizable (Fig. 25–1). If there is dilated bowel, usually at least 2 centimeters, it is important to recognize that the small bowel has folds extending all the way across it, known as the valvulae conniventes (Fig. 25–2). The colon, on the other hand, has folds that only partly extend across it, which are called the haustra (Fig. 25–3). If the entire bowel is dilated to a similar degree, then a paralytic ileus is present. If there is a discrepancy between small and large bowel dilatation, then mechanical obstruction is likely (Fig. 25–4), which is a surgical condition. If both sides of the bowel wall can be seen, then free air is present. Free intraperitoneal air frequently outlines the falciform ligament, and abnormal lucency is seen over the liver also (Fig. 25–5).

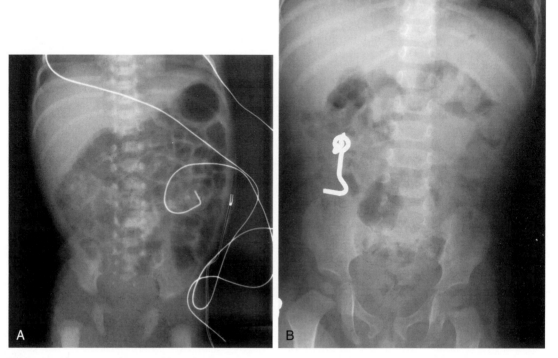

Figure 25–1. A, Normal neonatal bowel gas pattern in which small and large bowel are indistinguishable. **B,** Older patient with normal bowel gas pattern except for the ingested foreign body. Mainly only colon is seen.

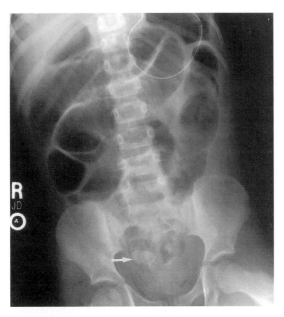

Figure 25–2. Dilated small bowel as diagnosed by the valvulae conniventes secondary to appendicitis with a large appendicolith seen in the pelvis *(arrow)*.

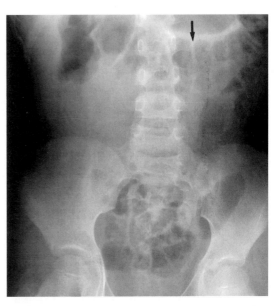

Figure 25–3. Haustra *(arrow)* seen in the colon in another patient with appendicitis.

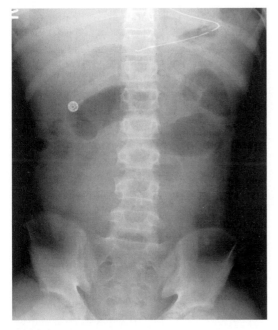

Figure 25–4. Small bowel obstruction is shown by the discrepancy between small bowel visualization and almost no colonic visualization.

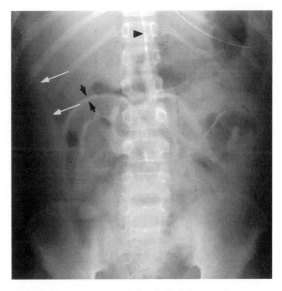

Figure 25–5. Free intraabdominal air in a supine person is demonstrated by the visualization of both sides of the bowel wall *(black arrows)*, outlining of the falciform ligament *(arrowhead)*, and abnormal lucency over the liver *(white arrows)*.

Calcifications

The most common calcifications are related to the biliary tract and the urinary tract and should be looked for in these locations. In addition, calcifications in the right lower quadrant (Fig. 25–2) could be due to fecaliths (i.e., appendicoliths). However, they are only present in a small percentage of patients with appendicitis. Other calcifications common to adults, such as vascular calcifications, both arterial and venous, are rare in children and should not create any confusion.

Skeletal Abnormalities

Observe the bones for any congenital abnormality that might be linked to the patient's clinical process. For example, the skeletal changes of Down syndrome, such as "Mickey Mouse ears" pelvis, could be linked to an acquired cause of bowel obstruction. Adhesions could have resulted from previous surgery for duodenal atresia, which is common in Down syndrome.

Evidence of previous trauma such as fractures, especially if found in the lumbar spine, could be indicative of underlying bowel injury (Fig. 25–6). This type of fracture is called chance fracture, where the fracture line runs through the vertebral body and posterior elements. This association is common in seat belt injuries in children usually younger than 8 years of age. Seat belt injuries can result in both lumbar spine fractures and bowel injury.

In older infants and children, the ossification of the spine is complete so that any congenital abnormality such as spina bifida changes should be obvious. With spina bifida, these changes consist of abnormal widening of the lumbar interpediculate distance and narrowing of the pedicles in the transverse dimension. Other vertebral anomalies may indicate underlying spinal cord abnormality as well (Fig. 25–7). Patients with spinal cord abnormality may have constipation as a result of their neurological impairment, which could lead to abdominal pain.

Organomegaly

Splenomegaly causes the stomach shadow to be pushed to the midline and pushes the splenic

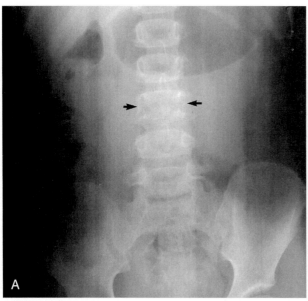
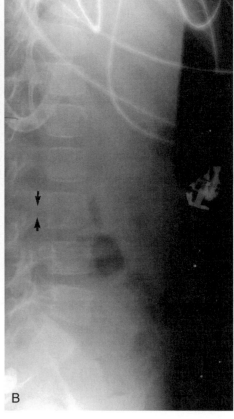

Figure 25–6. A, Chance fracture as demonstrated by apparent elongation of the pedicles *(arrows)* due to a fracture through them. **B,** Lateral view confirming the fracture through the posterior elements *(arrows).* The vertebral body fracture associated is less well seen.

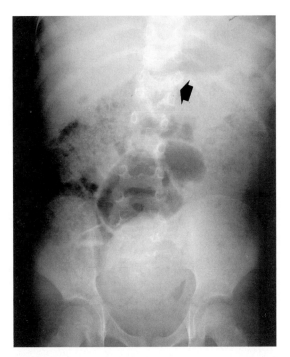

Figure 25–7. Patient with constipation due to spinal cord tethering. The vertebral anomaly *(arrow)* at T12 was the clue to the underlying cord abnormality demonstrated on subsequent MRI examination.

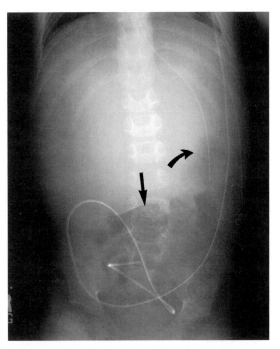

Figure 25–8. Hepatomegaly due to hepatoblastoma causing the transverse colon to be pushed inferiorly *(straight arrow)* and the stomach to be displaced toward the patient's left *(curved arrow).*

flexure of the colon inferiorly and toward the midline as well (Fig. 26–25). Hepatomegaly is easier to diagnose clinically than radiographically. There is a normal variant of the right lobe of the liver called a Reidel lobe that can simulate an enlarged liver. If the liver shadow extends to the iliac crest and displaces the bowel inferiorly and medially, then it probably is greatly enlarged (Fig. 25–8). Other enlarged organs in the abdomen can be seen, but the findings are much more subtle and are best evaluated by other imaging modalities.

Tubes, Catheters, Etc.

Vascular catheters, enteric tubes, and bladder catheters are the most commonly seen tubes in the abdomen. Without a lateral view or contrast material through these catheters, their position can only be inferred by where they project over known structures of the abdomen and pelvis. An enteric tube may actually be in a transpyloric location if the tip projects across the midline and points down inferiorly on a frontal view. However, a lateral view can help to confirm the position of the tube if it projects posteriorly, since the duodenum is a posterior structure. If no tube is

seen in the abdomen, inspection of the chest could reveal an aberrantly placed enteric tube (Fig. 25–9). Assessment of extraabdominal shadows should also be made. Body cast material, if applied too tightly, can result in acute abdominal pain due to acute superior mesenteric artery compression syndrome (Fig. 25–10). This causes obstruction

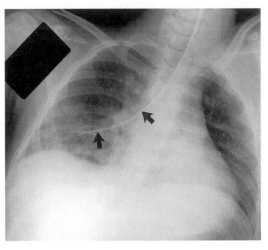

Figure 25–9. Aberrant placement of nasogastric tube into the right main stem bronchus *(arrows).*

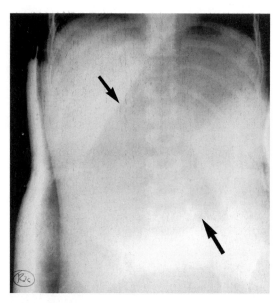

Figure 25–10. Cast syndrome causing massive gastric distension *(arrows)*. Cast syndrome is an acquired type of superior mesenteric artery compression syndrome.

at the second/third duodenal junction between the superior mesenteric artery and the aorta. This is also known as cast syndrome. A similar phenomenon can happen in patients who have lost a lot of weight or who have recently had scoliosis surgery.

MEDICAL CAUSES OF ABDOMINAL PAIN

Constipation

Constipation is a leading cause of chronic abdominal pain in the pediatric age group. Physical examination usually reveals large masses that represent fecal boluses. A single supine film is sometimes used to confirm the presence or absence of constipation (Fig. 25–11). The radiograph shows a bubbly appearance to the soft-tissue masses seen in the distribution of the colon. Chronic constipation rarely causes a small bowel obstruction. It is essential to evaluate the sacrum on these plain films to make sure that there is no sacral dysraphism (i.e., spina bifida) that might indicate that the constipation is due to an underlying neurologic abnormality. Other sacral anomalies may indicate previous surgery for an imperforate anus. These patients can have constipation as a complication of the pull-through procedure. In those cases in which a complication of the surgery is suspected, MRI is performed to evaluate the pelvic muscula-

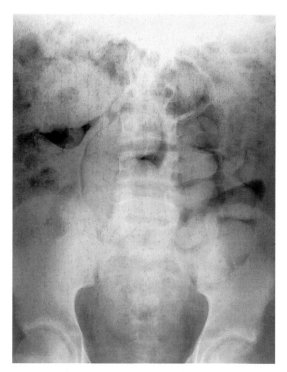

Figure 25–11. Abdominal film showing typical charges of constipation with fecal boluses throughout the expected location of the colon.

ture, specifically the levator ani muscle (Fig. 25–12). MRI can see if the musculature is present or if the placement of the new anus is correct. If the constipation has caused great dilatation to the underlying rectum, patients should have an evaluation for Hirschsprung syndrome, usually with a contrast enema. On occasion, Hirschsprung syndrome will present outside of the neonatal period (Fig. 25–13).

A special type of constipation occurs in patients suffering from cystic fibrosis. This has been called meconium ileus equivalent syndrome or distal intestinal obstruction syndrome (DIOS). The obstruction is due to the tenacious nature of the fecal stream in a patient with cystic fibrosis. The condition can be treated by enema, usually with hypertonic solutions that help to draw water into the stool, or by the ingestion of hyperosmolar agents that result in the same effect as the enema. Note: Older cystic fibrosis patients who once received high-dose pancreatic enzymes may actually have a surgical cause of abdominal pain. These patients are at risk for a colonic stricture because of the high doses of pancreatic enzymes that have been used in the past but are used in much smaller doses today.

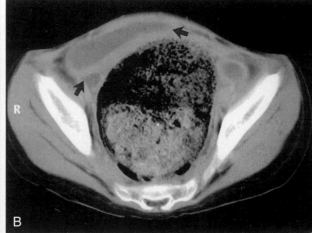

Figure 25–12. Axial T1-weighted image of the pelvic musculature in a patient with previous surgery for imperforate anus. Note the asymmetry of the levator ani on the left *(arrow)*, which presumably resulted from infarction of the muscle.

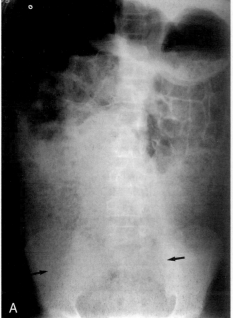

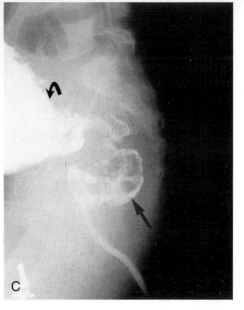

Figure 25–13. Hirschsprung syndrome seen in three different patients. **A,** Abdomen film of 13-year-old male showing massively dilated rectum *(arrows)* with a large amount of stool. **B,** CT of 12-year-old female with bladder outlet obstruction *(arrows)* secondary to large stool-filled rectum. **C,** Enema of 6-year-old showing typical transition zone between the spastic aganglionic segment *(straight arrow)* and the dilated more proximal normal colon *(curved arrow)*.

151

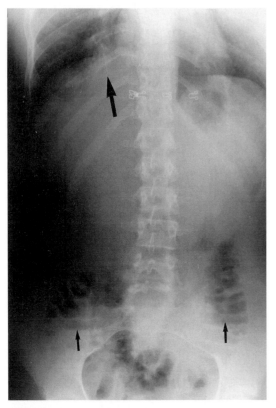

Figure 25–14. Patient with right lower lobe pneumonia *(large arrow)* who had an ileus with numerous air-filled levels in the colon *(small arrows)*. The patient had a normal appendix at surgery.

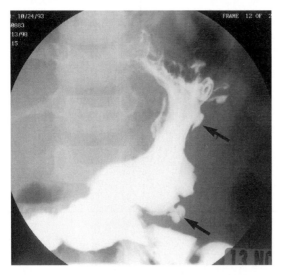

Figure 25–15. Patient with very large gastric folds and ulcers *(arrows)* secondary to severe peptic ulcer disease confirmed at endoscopy.

Gastroenteritis

Gastroenteritis is also a leading cause of abdominal pain in the pediatric age group. If radiographs are obtained, they can show dilated small and large bowel to the same degree (a paralytic ileus) with multiple air-fluid levels present on an upright examination, particularly in the colon. Air-fluid levels are not specific for gastroenteritis, but they are not normal in the colon. (Patients who recently have had an enema can also have air-fluid levels in the colon.) Other causes for an ileus pattern include metabolic disturbances, sepsis, and pancreatitis, among others. Beware of the patient with right lower lobe pneumonia who has referred pain to the abdomen (Fig. 25–14).

Peptic Ulcer Disease and Gastritis

Occasionally, children suffer from peptic ulcer disease and gastritis. These entities are more commonly seen in the adolescent population than in the younger child. Patients who are taking systemic steroid medication are also at risk for these conditions. The diagnosis is frequently inferred when the symptoms get better with antacid medication. If confirmatory evidence is needed, then

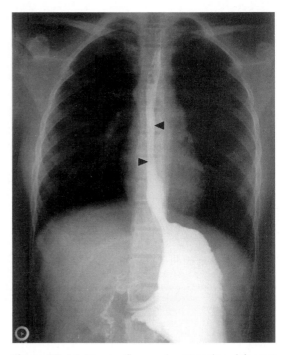

Figure 25–16. Severe reflux esophagitis in this adolescent causing a long, irregular esophageal stricture *(arrowheads)*.

the patient can have endoscopy or a barium upper gastrointestinal (UGI) series. Gastritis is difficult to diagnose on an UGI series, but an ulcer shows a persistent barium pocket with thickened gastric folds (Fig. 25–15). In addition, the duodenal folds are usually thickened. Observation for gastroesophageal reflux can also be completed at the time of the UGI series. Occasionally reflux is a cause of abdominal pain; however, it more commonly causes chest pain (Fig. 25–16).

Inflammatory Bowel Disease

Inflammatory bowel disease, regional enteritis and ulcerative colitis, starts to be an important cause of abdominal pain, particularly in the adolescent. Regional enteritis, Crohn disease, is usually diagnosed in patients over 10 years of age. The process can involve any portion of the intestinal tract, but most commonly it is seen in the terminal ileum (Fig. 25–17). It involves the entire wall of the intestine and causes the terminal ileum

to appear to stand out from the rest of the intestine because of the inflammation both in and around the involved bowel. Frequently there is also stricture formation and fistula formation in patients who have this entity. Diagnosis is suggested on an UGI series that also includes a view of the entire small bowel all the way to the colon, that is, small bowel follow-through.

Ulcerative colitis is occasionally seen in the pediatric age group and is limited to the colon. It is simply a mucosal process and is best assessed on an air-barium enema, that is, air-contrast BE (Fig. 25–18). The mucosa, which is normally featureless, is seen as little ulcers in the areas of involvement. The process starts from the rectum and ascends more proximally in a continuous fashion. Diagnosis is usually confirmed at colonoscopy.

Lymphoid nodular hyperplasia (LNH) is a normal finding in the pediatric population that can simulate inflammatory bowel disease. In the terminal ileum, it has a nodular appearance, but the

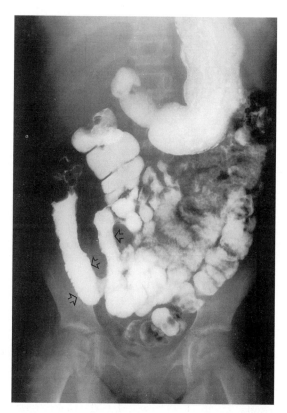

Figure 25–17. Crohn disease with involvement of the distal ileum *(open arrows)*. The involved loops are standing apart from the rest of the small bowel because of the transmural involvement of the inflammation.

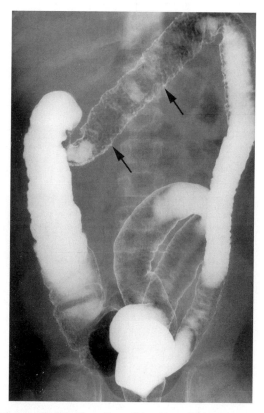

Figure 25–18. Ulcerative colitis with multiple tiny ulcers *(arrows)* seen on this air-contrast barium enema throughout the colon.

bowel is pliable and mobile with compression applied to it. In the colon, LNH has the appearance of little rounded areas with central barium-filled umbilications. Occasionally, bloody stools can be seen in the setting of LNH. The relationship between LNH and bloody stools is unknown. However, LNH should not be mistaken for the ulcerations seen in ulcerative colitis.

In a patient with abdominal pain a view of the chest is frequently obtained as part of a three-way view of the abdomen. The reason for the chest radiograph is to exclude a lower lobe pneumonia that might be causing referred pain into the abdomen. If the lower aspect of the chest is seen on the abdominal radiograph, it is important to scan the lower lobes on these films (Fig. 25–14). Because the technique of the abdominal film is darker than the chest film technique, the lung bases are best seen on this film, if they are included.

Pancreatitis

One third of cases of pancreatitis in the pediatric population are due to trauma. In those patients with pseudocysts especially, nonaccidental trama (i.e., child abuse) should be considered. Other causes of pancreatitis can include medications, hereditary types, and idiopathic etiology. The best imaging modality for pancreatitis is ultrasound. Frequently the pancreas is enlarged and is less echoic than the adjacent liver. Complications such as pseudocyst can be imaged first with CT and then followed with ultrasound when present (Fig. 25–19).

SURGICAL CAUSES OF ABDOMINAL PAIN

Small Bowel Obstruction

Once again, plain radiographs are usually the first imaging modality used in the evaluation of abdominal pain. Surgical conditions are those that show evidence of a bowel obstruction on plain radiographs. Bowel obstruction is demonstrated by the presence of a discrepancy between large and small bowel dilatation. If the condition has gone on long enough, the bowel loops assume a stacking appearance (Fig. 25–20). The more proximal the obstruction, the fewer dilated small bowel loops are seen.

The three most common causes of a small bowel obstruction (SBO) pattern (small bowel loops dilated out of proportion to the colon) in infants and children are intussusception, incarcerated inguinal hernia, and appendicitis. Other causes are adhesions from previous surgery, malrotation with Ladd bands and/or volvulus, among other less common entities.

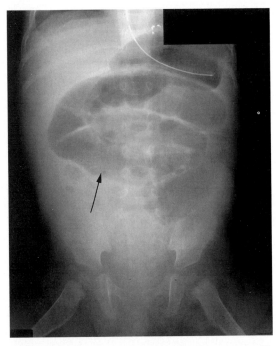

Figure 25–20. Small bowel obstruction pattern with "stacking" of loops of bowel. The valvulae conniventes (arrow) can be seen, which identify the loops as small bowel. There is essentially no colonic air.

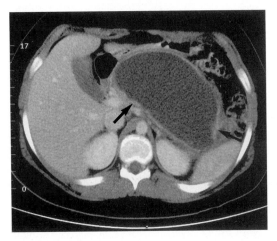

Figure 25–19. Patient with hereditary pancreatitis and resultant pseudocyst (arrows).

Intussusception

Intussusception is the most common cause of small bowel obstruction in infants and children. It is an idiopathic condition in patients that are 3 months to 4 years of age. In addition, this entity is a seasonal condition that is more likely to be present when upper respiratory tract infections (URI) are common. Clinically, these patients may have had a history of URI approximately 1 month before presentation. The theory as to why intussusception may occur in these patients is that the URI is thought to result in stimulation of the immune system, including Peyer patches of the small intestine. As a result, the enlarged lymph areas then may be a source of a "lead point" in the ileum that then intussuscepts into the colon. The most common type is, therefore, ileocolic. There is rarely a true lead point in these patients, but when there is one, it is usually a polyp or Meckel diverticulum. Those patients who have recurring episodes or are not in the typical age range for the idiopathic variety should be evaluated for a lead point. In the patient 6 years old or older with intussusception, the lead point is considered lymphoma until proven otherwise.

The initial imaging is usually a supine abdominal radiograph and left-side-down decubitus view or upright abdomen. The latter examination is to exclude free intraperitoneal air. However, whether the plain films need to be done at all is controversial. When they are performed, certain findings suggest the diagnosis of intussusception: no gas in the right lower quadrant, a small bowel obstruction or not enough gas for a presumed crying and air swallowing toddler, or the presence of a soft-tissue mass that represents the intussusceptum (Fig. 25–21). If there is gas in the right lower quadrant on plain film, the diagnosis is usually ruled out. Regardless of what the plain film shows, if the clinical suspicion is there, the diagnosis should be made or excluded by some sort of imaging, usually an enema.

Ultrasound can be performed as a screening procedure in cases where the symptoms are not typical. The appearance of an intussusception on ultrasound is that of a "pseudokidney" or of a whirled appearance of bowel when seen in cross-section (Fig. 25–22). A few pediatric radiologists then use a water enema and ultrasound guidance to reduce the intussusception until the "pseudokidney" appearance is gone. Most radiologists, however, use a radiographic enema, either air or positive contrast, to reduce the process. The enema shows a filling defect with convex borders when an intussusception is present (Fig. 25–23). The filling defect is the intussusceptum, which is the bowel that is intussuscepting into the more distal bowel, the intussuscipiens. With the pressure of the contrast, this soft-tissue mass is pushed

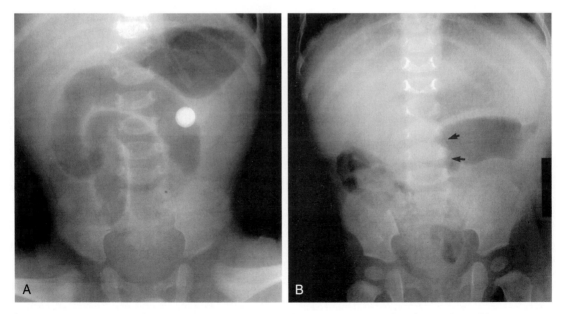

Figure 25–21. Two cases of intussusception: Small bowel obstruction pattern **(A)** and mass *(arrows)* intussusceptum on plain film **(B).**

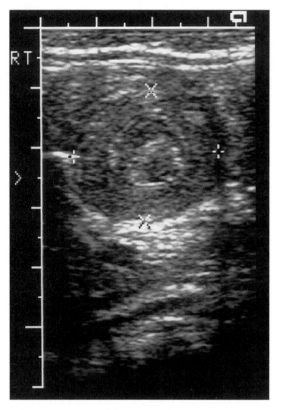

Figure 25–22. Ultrasound diagnosis of intussusception. The mass is measured by electronic calipers and has a "whirled" appearance in cross-section.

in a retrograde fashion back to the cecum and then into the ileum until the mass is no longer seen.

Incarcerated Inguinal Hernia

In boys, especially those less than 1 year of age, incarcerated inguinal hernia is a common cause of small bowel obstruction (Fig. 25–24). The diagnosis is usually made clinically, although ultrasound can be used to image bowel in the hernia sac. Contrast enemas are rarely used to visualize the bowel in the hernia. In patients in whom there is a question of hernia but not an incarcerated one and the physical examination is questionable, a herniagram can be performed. This study involves the infusion of either a radiographic contrast material or nuclear medicine radiopharmaceutical into the peritoneal cavity to see if the opening in the inguinal canal is present. When the hernia is present, the contrast agent will be seen in the scrotum.

Appendicitis

The diagnosis of appendicitis is usually a clinical one. When radiographs are performed, how-

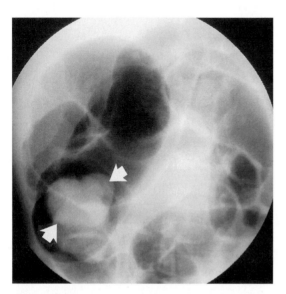

Figure 25–23. Air enema, which is used by most pediatric radiologists, has not completely reduced the intussusceptum *(arrows)* that is stuck at the ileocecal valve.

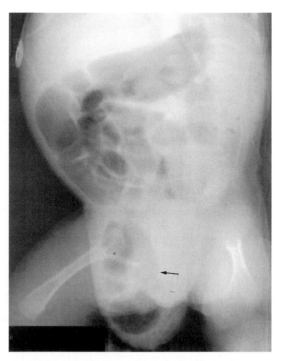

Figure 25–24. Right-sided inguinal hernia containing air-filled bowel *(arrow)*. Bowel distension in the abdomen is due to early obstruction of the hernia.

ever, the SBO pattern may be present. These patients are not usually obstructed unless there is a perforation with inflammatory tissue that is physically obstructing the bowel. Usually the reason for the SBO pattern is that of an ileus localized to the small bowel. However, it is once again the discrepancy of small bowel dilatation without colon dilatation that makes this a surgical condition by plain radiographs.

Other things to look for on the plain radiograph when the suspicion of appendicitis is present are absence of gas in the right lower quadrant, calcification usually in the right lower quadrant (Fig. 25–25) or right hemipelvis that represents an appendicolith (present in only 10 to 15 percent), abnormal bubbly gas pattern in the right lower quadrant that represents abscess formation from a perforated appendix, and infrequently, free intraperitoneal air from a perforated appendix.

When the diagnosis is in doubt and the plain films are not helpful, ultrasound is the modality of choice to visualize the appendix. The findings in appendicitis on ultrasound are those of a sausage-shaped mass in the right lower quadrant that is noncompressible with the ultrasound transducer and measures 6 millimeters or greater in transverse dimension (Fig. 25–26A and B). Sometimes appendicoliths are seen on ultrasound

(Fig. 25–26C). These calcifications are echogenic and block the ultrasound beam, which causes an acoustic shadow behind them. In addition, there may be a fluid collection in the right lower quadrant in the cases of appendiceal perforation.

A few institutions still perform contrast enema studies in these questionable cases. The radiographic criteria for the diagnosis of appendicitis are that of a mass effect on the cecum, caused by those cases associated with perforation and abscess formation, and absence of filling of the appendix. Obviously, a lot of cases of appendicitis do not have abscess formation, so looking for mass effect is not a sensitive way to evaluate for appendicitis. Absence of filling of the appendix has now been shown to occur in at least 10 percent of normal people, so this is also not a good criterion for the diagnosis. Even in those patients in whom the appendix fills, it may not be completely filled by contrast, and the appendix may only be inflamed at the tip. Therefore, because of the difficulties associated with the contrast enema in making the diagnosis of appendicitis, this modality has fallen out of favor with most radiologists.

CT scan of the abdomen with both intravenous and oral contrast material can also be used to diagnose appendicitis or an abscess associated with the appendicitis or both. To diagnose appen-

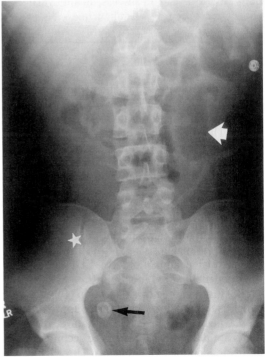

Figure 25–25. Plain film diagnosis of appendicitis: absence of gas in right lower quadrant *(star)*, dilated small bowel *(white arrow)*, and calcification in the right hemipelvis *(black arrow)*.

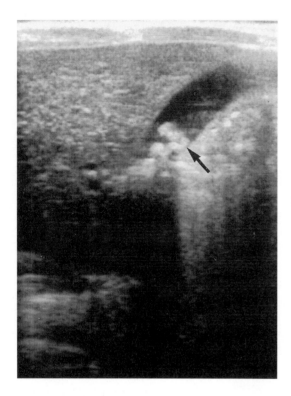

Figure 25–29. Typical case of gallstones *(arrow).*

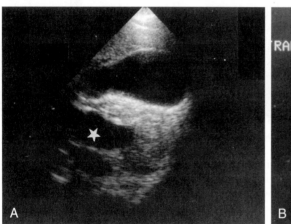

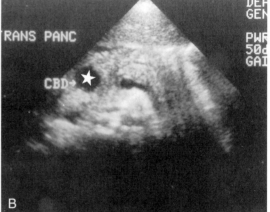

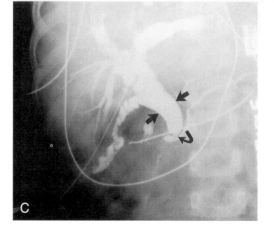

Figure 25–30. Choledochal cyst (type 1). **A,** Longitudinal view of gallbladder with dilated common bile duct seen below *(star).* **B,** Transverse view of dilated common bile duct *(star).* **C,** Intraoperative cholangiogram showing the dilated common bile duct *(straight arrows)* with its anomalous insertion into the pancreatic duct *(curved arrow).*

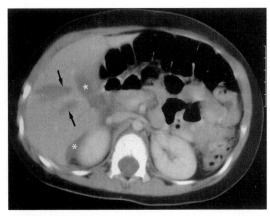

Figure 25–31. Liver laceration as shown by the hypoattenuation area *(arrows)* in the liver next to the gallbladder *(star)*. A small amount of free fluid is seen adjacent to the right kidney *(asterisk)*.

triad of abdominal mass, jaundice, and pain is rarely present. Ultrasound is the best imaging modality (Fig. 25–30).

Trauma to the abdomen can lead to abdominal pain. Damage to major organs can best be seen on a CT scan in the acute setting (Fig. 25–31). Ultrasound is best used in following known injuries. When imaging the abdomen by CT in suspected trauma, intravenous contrast is always needed unless the patient has renal compromise.

Oral contrast is not usually needed because the pediatric patient frequently has an ileus and the contrast sits in the stomach. Air is then used as the bowel contrast. Rectal contrast is only given in children when there is a history of penetrating injury in the pelvic area.

Occasionally obstructive uropathy can result in diffuse abdominal pain. Abdominal ultrasound can detect the abnormality followed by nuclear medicine renogram as discussed in other chapters.

Chapter 26

The Older Infant and Child with an Abdominal Mass

Ultrasound is the imaging modality of choice in a patient with a suspected abdominal mass. It is the best and cheapest screening modality, and it involves no radiation. Once a mass has been diagnosed, then other imaging modalities can be used, with CT being the most common. MRI has limited value in abdominal mass imaging because of the motion artifact from the gut. However, it is of value in retroperitoneal tumors that might invade the spinal cord.

RETROPERITONEAL MASSES OF RENAL ORIGIN

In the older infant and child, as in the neonate, retroperitoneal tumors are the most common abdominal masses. Fifty-five percent of the time they are renal in origin with Wilms tumor and hydronephrosis being the most common.

Wilms Tumor

Wilms tumor arises from the kidney and is the most common malignant abdominal neoplasm in children from 1 to 8 years of age. The peak age for Wilms tumor is 3 years. It is usually unilateral (Fig. 26–1) but is bilateral in approximately 10 percent of cases. There are underlying syndromes that are commonly associated with Wilms tumor. Patients with these syndromes need periodic screening. The syndromes include Beckwith-Wiedemann syndrome (macroglossia, organomegaly, omphalocele); sporadic aniridia (hypoplasia of iris); hemihypertrophy (one side of the body is bigger than the other); and Drash syndrome (Fig. 26–2) (ambiguous genitalia, bilateral Wilms, and nephrotic syndrome). Patients with renal anomalies like horseshoe kidney or other fusion anomaly of the kidney are also at risk for developing Wilms tumor.

Imaging. Imaging of Wilms tumor starts with ultrasound, which usually shows a fairly homogeneous hyperechoic mass that arises from the kidney. Because there is a propensity for Wilms tumor to invade the inferior vena cava, ultrasound

is the chief imaging modality to screen for this process. Chest radiograph is performed to evaluate for chest metastases. CT is then done to evaluate for distant metastases such as in the liver and lymph nodes in the retroperitoneum. If the chest radiograph is negative for metastases, chest CT is usually not performed. The tumor itself arises from the kidney and is seen to cause calyceal distortion. It is often huge (Fig. 26–3) and sometimes causes an anterior abdominal wall contour defect. Calcification in Wilms tumor only occurs 10 to 15 percent of the time. MRI is not usually used in the evaluation of Wilms tumor but can be when the question of inferior vena cava invasion cannot be answered with ultrasound (Fig. 26–4).

Hydronephrosis

Hydronephrosis is another cause for an abdominal mass in the older infant and child. Hydronephrosis can be caused by vesicoureteral reflux and obstruction. The obstruction can be at the level of the renal pelvis (ureteropelvic junction [UPJ]), at the bladder (ureterovesical junction [UVJ]), or

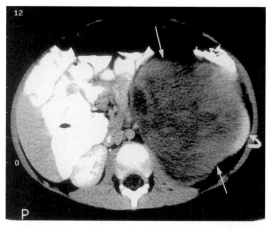

Figure 26–1. Large left-sided Wilms tumor *(straight arrows)* that is inhomogeneous in enhancement because of its large size. There is a tiny rim of normal kidney seen laterally *(curved arrow)*, confirming that the mass is of renal origin.

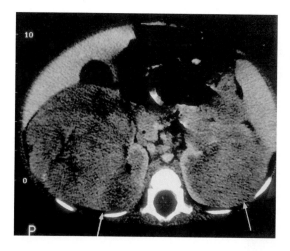

Figure 26–2. Bilateral Wilms tumors *(arrows)* in a patient with Drash syndrome.

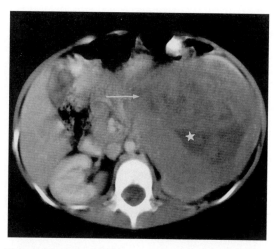

Figure 26–3. Huge Wilms tumor that extends to the midline *(arrow)* and has areas of necrosis *(star)* within it because of its large size. A remnant of normal renal tissue is seen anteriorly.

Figure 26–4. Large renal tumor *(wide arrows)* that was seen to compress the inferior vena cava *(thin arrow)*. Frozen section diagnosis was Wilms tumor, but final histology was peripheral neuroectodermal tumor *(PNET)*.

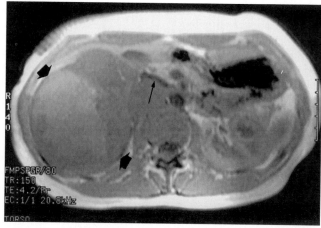

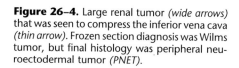

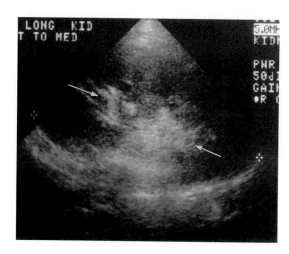

Figure 26–5. Normal renal ultrasound in an older child. The collecting system echoes are seen centrally as increased echogenicity *(arrows)*.

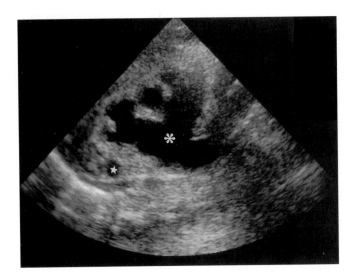

Figure 26–6. Hydronephrotic lower pole system *(asterisk)* as demonstrated by the echolucent area. The upper pole is quite small *(star)* in this duplicated system.

at the distal ureter (distal adynamic segment of ureter). In addition, only a portion of the kidney can be obstructed, as is seen with a completely duplicated collecting system that has an obstructed upper renal pole.

Imaging. Imaging of hydronephrosis is best done with ultrasound. The normal renal ultrasound in the older child shows that there is no longer prominence of the medullary pyramids as in the neonate (Fig. 26–5). The renal cortex becomes less echoic than the adjacent liver and spleen in patients older than about 1 year of age. The normal collecting system echo complex is echogenic diffusely without echolucency seen in the center. When there are two sets of calyceal echoes, a duplicated system is suspected (Fig. 26–6).

In hydronephrosis, the collecting system echo complex is separated by lucency that represents urine in a dilated collecting system. If the system is completely duplicated, the upper pole is classically obstructed and frequently associated with an ectopic ureterocele (a bulbous dilatation of the distal ureter that enters ectopically) and the lower pole usually refluxes. Therefore, both collecting system echo complexes can show separation for different reasons. Intravenous urography, also known as intravenous pyelography (IVP), is no longer routinely used for renal imaging (Fig. 26–7). It is still used to demonstrate ureteral abnormality such as the location of ectopic ureteric insertions.

Views of the bladder are always obtained when the kidneys are imaged. Dilated ureters are frequently seen at the level of the bladder. In addition, ureteroceles can be observed inside the bladder (Fig. 26–8). If a dilated ureter is seen, as well as hydronephrosis, the appearance is consistent with vesicoureteral reflux, ureterovesical obstruction, or distal adynamic segment of the ureter.

Once hydronephrosis is diagnosed on ultrasound, the next imaging procedure should be a voiding cystourethrogram (VCUG) (Fig. 26–9). This study will determine whether reflux is present.

If no reflux is present as a cause of hydronephrosis, then a nuclear medicine renogram is in

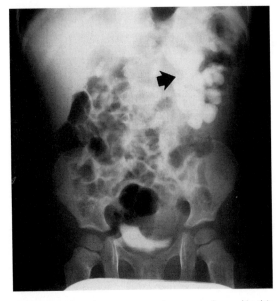

Figure 26–7. An intravenous pyelogram performed in this patient with ureteropelvic junction obstruction *(arrow).*

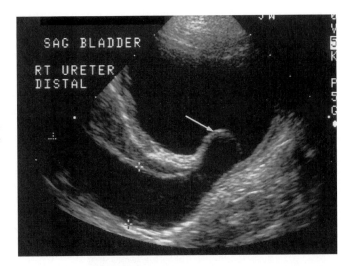

Figure 26–8. Demonstration of ureterocele with a bulbous end *(arrow)* entering into the bladder.

order. The renogram can determine whether obstruction is present and how much renal function the hydronephrotic kidney has. This study involves monitoring the intravenous injection of a radiopharmaceutical that is taken up by the kidney and excreted. Usually a diuretic (furosemide) is given during the examination to enhance excretion. Computer-generated curves of this activity are achieved. This study is a functional study of the kidney that will show whether or not a system is obstructed (Fig. 26–10).

RETROPERITONEAL MASSES OF NONRENAL ORIGIN

Nonrenal retroperitoneal masses make up 25 percent of abdominal masses, with neuroblastoma being the most common.

Neuroblastoma

Neuroblastoma is seen in children who are slightly younger than the age range for Wilms

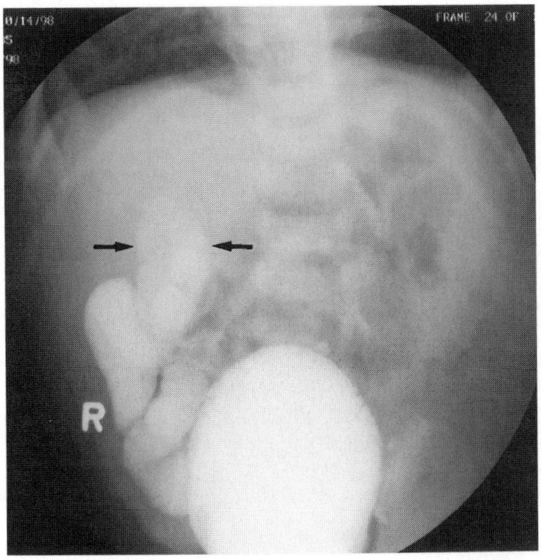

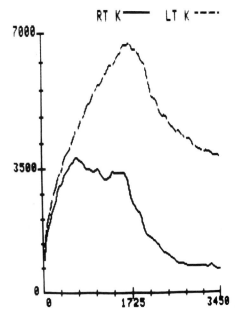

Figure 26–9. Massive vesicoureteral reflux on right during voiding cystourethrogram *(arrows)*. Ultrasound showed hydronephrosis, which was due to reflux and not obstruction.

Figure 26–10. Renal function curves from furosemide renogram. The up slope of the curve is when the kidney takes up the radiopharmaceutical. The downward slope indicates excretion and not obstruction. Here the right kidney has less function than the left.

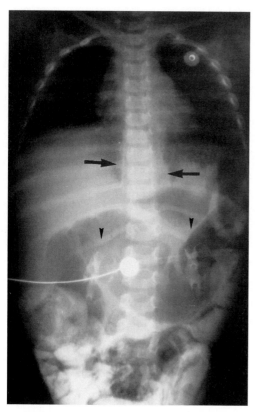

Figure 26–11. Radiograph obtained after CT scan shows adenopathy *(arrows)* along paraspinous region and displacement of both kidneys inferiorly *(arrowheads)* by neuroblastoma.

tumor, but there is an overlap of these age ranges. When neuroblastoma is discovered in the abdomen, it is usually widespread and unresectable at the time of diagnosis.

Imaging. On imaging, ultrasound usually shows a more heterogeneously echoic mass than Wilms tumor. Seventy-five to eighty percent of the time there is calcification and hemorrhage within it. The mass usually pushes the kidney around rather than distort it (Fig. 26–11). With CT, the tumor is seen to encase and distort the position of the inferior vena cava and aorta (Fig. 26–12). The tumor crosses the midline and frequently has metastases in the liver at the time of diagnosis. Besides metastases to lymph nodes and liver, neuroblastoma frequently goes to bones and causes lytic lesions. Skeletal survey and nuclear medicine bone scanning are complimentary imaging modalities for evaluating skeletal metastases. Lesions that are lytic are best appreciated on skeletal survey. Bone scanning can help in the preoperative diagnosis because the soft-tissue component of the tumor takes up the radiopharmaceutical in over two thirds of the cases.

OTHER MASSES

Genital Masses

Genital masses are less commonly a cause of abdominal mass in the older infant and child than in the neonate. These masses make up only approximately 5 percent of the total and are mostly ovarian cysts and teratomas. Teratomas can arise

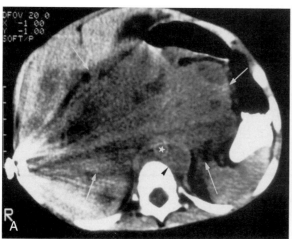
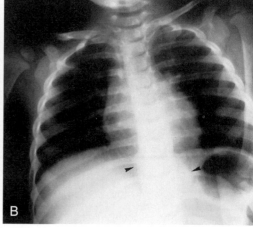

Figure 26–12. A, Unenhanced CT scan showing huge mass *(arrows)* of neuroblastoma. The aorta *(star)* is surrounded by adenopathy *(arrowhead)*, which corresponds to the widened paraspinous line on the chest x-ray **(B)** *(arrowheads)*.

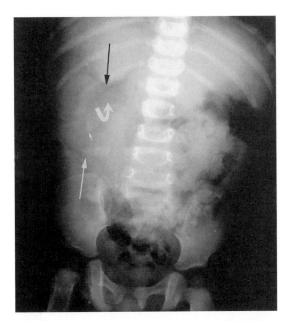

Figure 26–13. Plain abdominal film in a patient with a history of vomiting. An ill-defined mass was seen in the right upper quadrant *(long arrows)* that was confirmed on ultrasound and subsequent CT. Surgery confirmed the diagnosis of a retroperitoneal teratoma. The area of lucency represented fat *(curved arrow)*, and there were small calcifications *(short arrow)* present, as well.

from the retroperitoneum as well as the ovary (Fig. 26–13). Ultrasound is the imaging modality of choice, particularly when there is an ovarian cyst present. An uncomplicated cyst is anechoic and easily seen by using the full bladder as an acoustic window. A teratoma has mixed echogeni-

city to it due to the complex histologic makeup of the tumor. Fat and calcification, which are seen in the vast majority of teratomas, are echogenic. CT scan is performed on some teratomas to confirm their makeup (Fig. 26–14).

Gastrointestinal Masses

Gastrointestinal masses account for approximately 10 percent of the abdominal masses in the older infant and child. Stool is most often the cause for the "mass" (Fig. 26–15). Other entities in the differential diagnosis include abscess (usually from a perforated appendix), intussusception (Fig. 26–16), hepatobiliary masses such as hepatomegaly from an infectious etiology and hepatic neoplasm, choledochal cyst, pancreatic mass such as pancreatic pseudocyst, and splenic mass usually due to splenomegaly from either an infectious etiology or from a neoplastic cause.

Appendiceal Abscess. Abscess from a perforated appendix can be suggested from the plain abdominal radiograph, as there are unusual bubbly gas lucencies in the right lower quadrant. In addition, if there is an appendicolith seen on the radiograph in a symptomatic patient, the incidence of appendiceal perforation is high (Fig. 26–17). Abdominal ultrasound is the imaging modality of choice for the initial investigation of this entity if the plain radiographs and clinical symptoms are not characteristic. Abdominal CT can be performed for confirmation or as an investigative tool in those patients that have an indeterminate ultrasound, but the clinical suspicion is

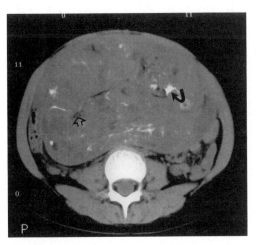

Figure 26–14. Large teratoma thought to be ovarian in origin shown to contain calcifications *(curved arrow)* and fat *(open arrow)* on unenhanced CT scan.

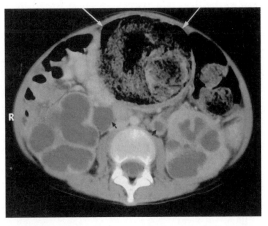

Figure 26–15. Large boluses of stool *(long arrows)* caused this patient's abdominal mass. The colon was so dilated from Hirschsprung syndrome that the ureters *(short arrows)* and kidneys were obstructed.

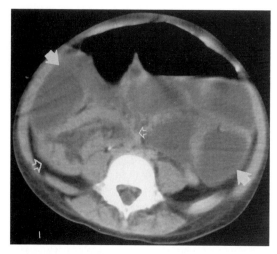

Figure 26–16. CT scan of intussusception showing mass in right lower quadrant *(open arrows)*. The scan was performed on this cancer patient to exclude a cause for obstruction versus ileus from chemotherapy that resulted in the dilated bowel loops *(closed arrows)*.

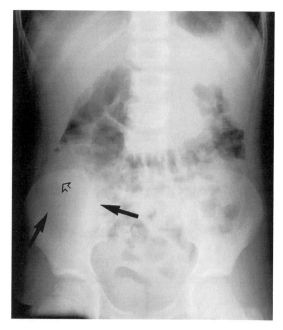

Figure 26–17. Perforated appendix with mass effect in the right lower quadrant *(closed arrows)* and subtle calcification from fecalith *(open arrow)*.

still high. CT scan can also help to diagnose complications of appendicitis such as liver abscess (Fig. 26–18).

Hepatomegaly. Hepatic enlargement can be due to hepatitis, which is usually suspected on clinical grounds because of elevation of hepatic enzymes. If imaging is employed, ultrasound can show the liver parenchyma to be decreased with the periportal and peribiliary echoes appearing more echoic than normal (Fig. 26–19). This appearance is not specific for hepatitis and is seen in any edematous state of the liver. Fatty infiltration of the liver can also cause an enlarged liver.

Since fat is echogenic on ultrasound, the liver is too echogenic, which obscures the underlying normal hepatic architecture. The liver is also hard to penetrate with ultrasound in these cases. On CT scan the liver has less attenuation than the spleen on unenhanced scans (Fig. 26–20). Usually, liver and spleen are equal in attenuation.

When the liver is enlarged because of neoplasm, metastasis is the most common, usually due to neuroblastoma metastases. Primary hepatic neoplasm in a child under age 5 years is usually

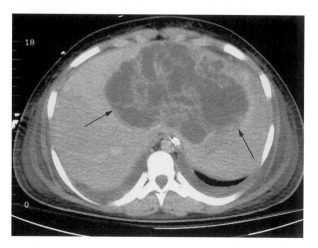

Figure 26–18. Liver abscess *(arrows)* from presumed perforated appendix.

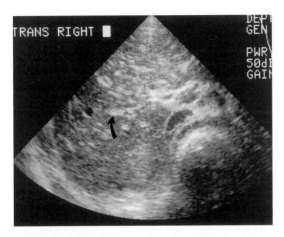

Figure 26–19. Transverse liver ultrasound showing increased periportal and biliary echoes *(arrow)* from hepatitis.

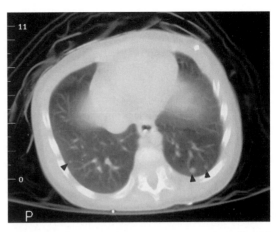

Figure 26–21. Hepatoblastoma metastases *(arrowheads)* seen on the lung base slices of an abdominal CT.

due to hepatoblastoma. Abdominal CT best evaluates this lesion as to possible resectability because the anatomy of the liver is best appreciated with this modality. Hepatoblastoma is calcified in approximately 25 to 30 percent of the cases and is moderately enhancing with intravenous contrast. Lung metastases are best appreciated with chest CT, as well (Fig. 26–21). Clinically, the alpha fetoprotein level is extremely high in the vast majority of the cases of hepatoblastoma. In the slightly older patient, hepatocellular carcinoma is the cause of a primary hepatic malignancy. The imaging features are similar, but the alpha fetoprotein is not elevated in as many cases.

Choledochal Cyst. Choledochal cyst can present as a right upper quadrant mass in the older child. Sometimes the patient has symptoms of pancreatitis and the cyst is seen on screening ultrasound (Fig. 26–22). Sometimes the cyst is seen when a screening abdominal CT (Fig. 26–23) for abdominal trauma is performed.

Pseudocyst. Pancreatic masses in children are not common, but a pseudocyst is the most frequently encountered mass. The cause of pancreatitis is trauma in at least one third of the cases, but when a pseudocyst is encountered, the incidence of traumatic origin increases. Ultrasound

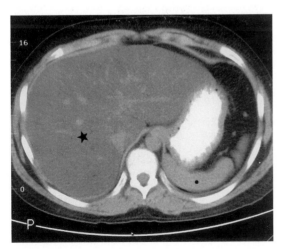

Figure 26–20. Fatty liver on CT with the liver of decreased attenuation *(star)* compared with the spleen *(asterisk)*.

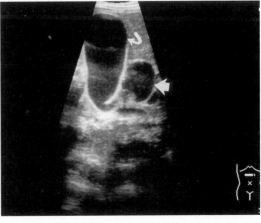

Figure 26–22. Choledochal cyst seen on ultrasound. The dilated common bile duct *(straight arrow)* is seen adjacent to the gallbladder *(curved arrow)*.

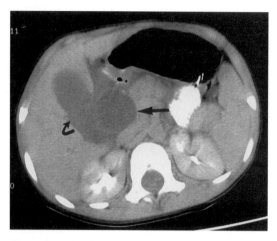

Figure 26–23. Choledochal cyst *(straight arrow)* on CT scan adjacent to the gallbladder *(curved arrow)*.

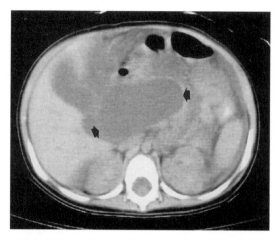

Figure 26–24. CT scan of patient with pancreatic pseudocyst *(arrows)* that was eventually drained endoscopically into the stomach.

is a good imaging modality for following pseudocysts, but CT (Fig. 26–24) is most useful early in the initial diagnosis since the pseudocysts can extend into a variety of locations that could be obscured by overlying gas, which would make ultrasound less sensitive for the diagnosis.

Splenomegaly. Splenomegaly can be due to an infectious agent, such as Epstein-Barr virus, to a neoplastic cause such as involvement with leukemia or lymphoma, or to a blood dyscrasia. Splenomegaly can be suspected on chest radiograph when the stomach is displaced medially (Fig. 26–25). Ultrasound is invaluable to make sure that the mass felt in the left upper quadrant is indeed spleen and to then make sure that the spleen is homogeneous in echogenicity. CT has little role in the evaluation of splenomegaly, except when lymphoma is the culprit, and then other areas of involvement with lymphoma can be evaluated with CT. With viral-induced splenomegaly or blood dyscrasia-induced splenomegaly, the echogenicity is uniform. Leukemia also characteristically causes uniform echogenicity, although it has been described as echolucent masses, which is identical to that reported when the spleen is involved with lymphoma.

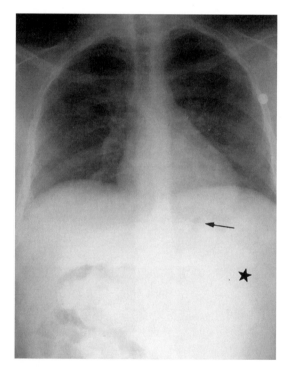

Figure 26–25. Splenomegaly *(star)* suspected on chest radiograph causing medial displacement of the stomach *(arrow)*.

Chapter 27

The Older Infant and Child with Guaiac-Positive or Frankly Bloody Stools

Causes of bloody stools are age related. In the younger patient, bleeding from a Meckel diverticulum, hyperplastic polyp, or from an intussusception are the three most common diagnoses that require imaging. In adolescents, although uncommon, inflammatory bowel disease and peptic ulcer disease are seen more frequently than in the younger, pediatric patient.

MECKEL DIVERTICULUM

These diverticula present in patients who are under 10 years of age. Most of them are seen in young children less than 2 years old. The diverticulum is a persistent remnant of the omphalomesenteric duct, which normally obliterates by the fifth fetal week. The vast majority of those that bleed contain gastric mucosa. The basis of imaging for the bleeding Meckel diverticulum is to look for the ectopic gastric mucosa contained in it by means of a nuclear medicine scan. Enteric duplication cysts can also present with bleeding, but usually symptoms are the result of mass effect (Fig. 27–1).

In this nuclear medicine examination the radiopharmaceutical is excreted by gastric mucosa. Therefore, after the radiopharmaceutical is injected, activity is sought in an ectopic location to appear at the same time as regular stomach activity. This location is usually in the right lower quadrant, although it can appear elsewhere (Fig. 27–2).

Barium or other radiopaque contrast agents have no role in this diagnosis since the diverticula rarely fill with the contrast. In fact, barium in the abdomen can block the activity from the radiopharmaceutical, preventing it from reaching the gamma camera. (Water-soluble contrast agents do not have this effect.)

INTUSSUSCEPTION

Intussusception, as discussed in Chapter 25, is usually diagnosed by an enema, usually an air

enema. Sometimes ultrasound is used for this diagnosis but only as a screening tool. The definitive diagnosis and treatment usually rests with the enema.

JUVENILE POLYPS

Juvenile polyps are the most common tumors of the colon in childhood. Some of the polyps are inflammatory, and some are hamartomas. Usually they are simple, large, and pedunculated and are located in the sigmoid colon or rectum. The symptoms are painless rectal bleeding in children who are usually between the ages of 2 and 10 years. They are most frequently diagnosed with colonoscopy. If imaging is needed, an air-contrast barium enema is the imaging procedure of choice. The enema needs to be performed after the colon has been evacuated because retained stool can simulate a polyp.

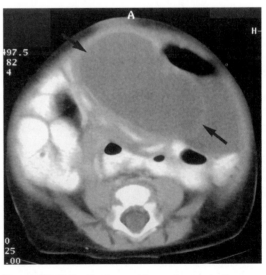

Figure 27–1. Duplication cyst *(arrows)* presented because a mass was felt in the abdomen.

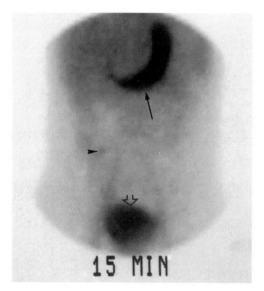

Figure 27–2. Positive Meckel diverticulum scan as seen on this 15-minute image. Stomach activity is in the upper abdomen *(long arrow)*, and bladder activity is at the bottom *(open arrow)*. The other area of increased activity is gastric mucosa within the Meckel diverticulum *(arrowhead)*.

PEPTIC ULCER DISEASE

With peptic ulcer disease, barium evaluation of the esophagus, stomach, and duodenum is sufficient. Although some patients are diagnosed by endoscopy, this barium examination is called an upper gastrointestinal tract study (UGI). Symptoms of peptic ulcer disease include thickened gastric and duodenal folds as well as demonstration of an ulcer crater with a persistent collection of barium in it (Fig. 27–3).

INFLAMMATORY BOWEL DISEASE

Inflammatory bowel disease is divided into two entities: Crohn disease and ulcerative colitis. The

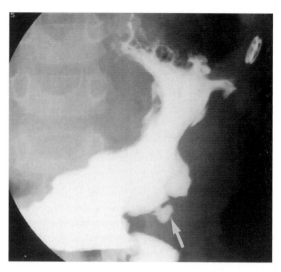

Figure 27–3. Patient with severe ulcer disease at endoscopy. The arrow shows a large ulcer crater.

latter diagnosis is uncommon in pediatrics. Pediatric patients with Crohn disease fail to thrive because of the malabsorption that this disease causes. As was discussed in Chapter 25, the diagnosis of Crohn disease rests with the upper gastrointestinal series and the small bowel follow-through, since the terminal ileum is usually the first location to be involved with the process. Findings with Crohn disease can range from a narrowed terminal ileum (string sign), to fistula formation, to diffuse bowel involvement showing thickened loops separated from the other bowel (Fig. 25–17).

With ulcerative colitis an air-contrast barium enema is the desired imaging tool. Only the colon is abnormal in this entity. The air-contrast barium enema shows small little ulcers along the colon, depending on the extent of involvement (Fig. 25–18).

Chapter 28

The Patient with a Febrile Urinary Tract Infection

Damage to the kidneys from infection, usually from reflux (reflux nephropathy), can have long-term, severe consequences. Hypertension is a common consequence of reflux nephropathy, and even renal failure can result. Therefore, all children with a documented febrile urinary tract infection should be evaluated, regardless of the sex of the patient.

In addition, at least one third of siblings of patients with vesicoureteral reflux have an increased incidence of reflux. Regardless of symptoms, a screening evaluation for siblings is also performed.

EVALUATION

Renal ultrasound and voiding cystourethrograms (VCUG) are the main imaging modalities performed on patients with a history of a febrile urinary tract infection. The VCUG is routinely performed in the patient who is no longer symptomatic. Frequently, the patient is on antibiotics at the time of the study. The ultrasound is usually performed in the acutely ill patient to observe for any obstruction that might need surgical drainage such as with ureteropelvic junction obstruction or an upper pole obstruction in a duplicated system.

In siblings of patients with vesicoureteral reflux, those with a history of infection are investigated similarly with at least an ultrasound and sometimes a VCUG. Siblings who are asymptomatic are investigated according to their age. Although the exact evaluation of siblings is controversial, the following age-related guidelines are frequently used. The younger siblings, less than 3 years of age, need both an ultrasound and VCUG. Girls in the age range of 3 to 5 years may need both procedures, but boys in this age range only need an ultrasound. Older siblings, regardless of sex, need only undergo an ultrasound. If the ultrasound is abnormal, a VCUG should be performed.

ULTRASOUND

Size of the kidney and gross renal scarring can be assessed on ultrasound. Reflux nephropathy most often involves the renal poles. The ultrasound shows scarring by demonstration of the calyceal echoes close to the edge of the kidney (Fig. 28–1). A small kidney can be due to reflux nephropathy as well.

On ultrasound, the presence or absence of pyelonephritis can sometimes be assessed. In the presence of clinical pyelonephritis, the kidney can

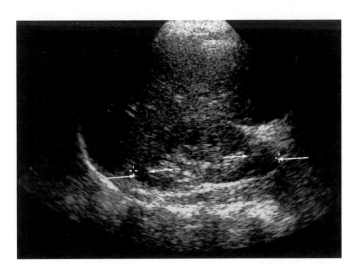

Figure 28–1. Reflux nephropathy with scarring in the upper pole. Note how the distance between the upper collecting system echoes and the edge of the kidney is smaller than the distance in the lower pole *(arrows)*.

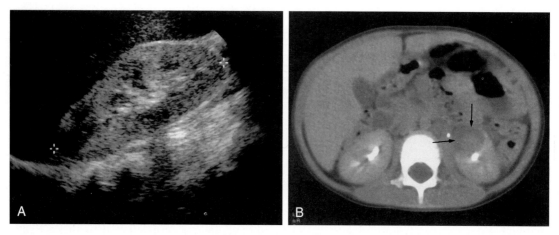

Figure 28–2. A, Echogenic kidney from infection. At this child's age (6 years), the kidney should be less echoic than the liver and spleen. In this patient the kidney is much more echogenic than the adjacent spleen. The kidney is demarcated by cursors. **B,** CT scan of same patient. A hypoattenuating area in the left kidney *(arrows)* was felt to represent abscess formation that was not appreciated at ultrasound.

look normal but can also appear enlarged with increased or decreased echogenicity (Fig. 28–2A). If the ultrasound is inconclusive and the patient is still febrile despite adequate therapy, CT scan may be performed to evaluate for renal abscess (Fig. 28–2B). Nuclear medicine, as stated below, can also be performed, although it involves a lot of radiation to the kidney.

In addition, the bladder should be imaged to evaluate for thickening of the wall and to observe for ureteral dilatation. Thickening of the bladder wall can occur with inflammation, neurogenic bladder, bladder-outlet obstruction, and, although rare, tumor involvement. Measurement of the bladder wall in the longitudinal plane must be done. For a distended bladder, 3 millimeters is the upper limit of normal. For a nondistended bladder, 5 millimeters is the upper limit of normal (Fig. 28–3).

Other findings on bladder sonography are the sonographic characteristics of the urine in the bladder. When a fluid-fluid level is encountered in the bladder, infection should be excluded. Likewise, if bladder stones are seen, infection should be considered. Infection should be suspected if any echogenic material is seen in the bladder urine.

At bladder sonography, a normal finding incidentally seen is the visualization of ureteral jets of urine as the urine empties normally from the ureters into the bladder. This finding can be seen with color Doppler.

VOIDING CYSTOURETHROGRAM

A VCUG needs to be performed in the asymptomatic patient. Historically, 6 weeks after the infection was the magic timing for the study. New data support performing the study earlier, because some patients will only demonstrate vesicoureteral reflux while inflammation is still present. At 6 weeks, the reflux may have resolved, and therefore the patient will be undertreated with antibiotic therapy.

In boys a fluoroscopic VCUG should be done (Fig. 28–4A). In girls, however, some centers advocate a nuclear medicine cystogram, since it gives less radiation to the female gonads. At most centers a fluoroscopic cystogram using pulsed fluoroscopy as well as digital imaging is done initially on all patients (Fig. 28–4B). Cyclic voiding is performed on younger children (usually those less than 1 year of age) when feasible. Cyclic voiding is when the contrast-filled bladder is emptied and then refilled during the examination. Those with reflux are then followed up with either nuclear medicine cystography or repeat fluoroscopic cystography.

Bladder volume, bladder configuration, and the presence or absence of vesicoureteral reflux are the most important pieces of information to gain from the VCUG. In addition, the presence of urethral pathology, especially in boys, is desired on the voiding phase of the study. Voiding is crucial regardless of the sex of the child, since it is only

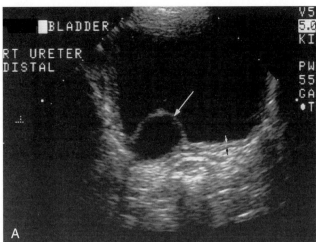

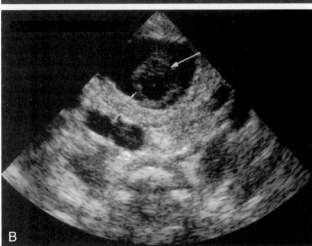

Figure 28–3. A, Bladder ultrasound showing ureterocele *(large arrow)* and the bladder wall *(small arrows)*. The wall should be measured on longitudinal midline image only. **B,** Another patient with a markedly thickened bladder *(small arrows)* and ureterocele *(large arrow)* that prolapsed into the urethra with voiding and caused bladder outlet obstruction.

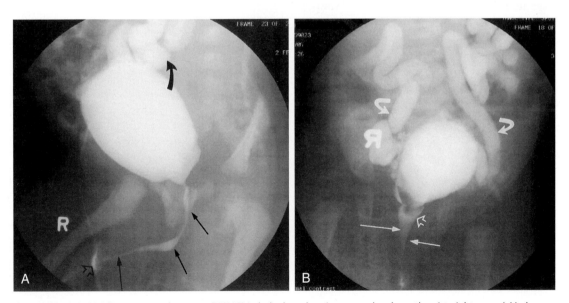

Figure 28–4. A, Voiding cystourethrogram (VCUG) in baby boy showing normal male urethra *(straight arrows)*. Vesicoureteral reflux, grade V, can be seen on the right *(curved arrow)*. At the tip of the urethra, a collection of contrast is seen that represents pooling of contrast in the foreskin *(open arrow)*. **B,** VCUG in baby girl with bilateral grade V reflux *(curved arrows)* and prolapsing ureterocele *(open arrow)* into bladder neck and female urethra *(straight arrows)*.

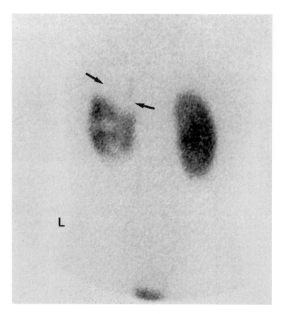

L

Figure 28–5. Renal scan in a patient with left-sided pyelo-nephritis showing photon deficient areas throughout the kidney, particularly the upper pole *(arrows)*.

at voiding that reflux occurs in some children. In addition, attaining maximal bladder capacity is also important since reflux sometimes only occurs at that volume.

Bladder volume is estimated according to the following formula:

(Age in years + 2) × 30 ml = Bladder volume

This formula is valid up to 14 years of age. Patients with abnormally large bladders are those with vesicoureteral reflux, infrequent voiders (those patients who have voided so infrequently for so long that their bladder capacity has increased over time), dysfunctional voiders (those patients who demonstrate abnormal perineal responses to voiding that increases the bladder pressures upon voiding), and patients with neurogenic bladders. Patients with large bladder volumes are at risk for infection because of the urine stasis that occurs.

As previously stated, vesicoureteral reflux is evaluated by using a 5-point grading system:

Grade 1 = Reflux into the ureter only
Grade 2 = Reflux extending up to the calyces without dilatation
Grade 3 = Reflux causing calyceal dilatation with slight ureteral dilatation
Grade 4 = Reflux causing both calyceal and ureteric dilatation as well as ureteral tortuosity
Grade 5 = Massive dilatation of the whole pelvocalyceal and ureteric system

NUCLEAR MEDICINE RENAL SCAN

If the diagnosis of pyelonephritis is in doubt, a nuclear medicine renal scan using a cortical labeling agent can be performed. Unfortunately the renal scan is expensive and involves giving the kidney a lot of radiation. On the scan, a photon-deficient area (Fig. 28–5) is seen in the acutely inflamed region that may or may not lead to renal scarring. The renal scan is performed mainly to evaluate for scarring and to clarify a puzzling ultrasound or unclear CT cases when there is a question of pyelonephritis.

Chapter 29

Accidental Skeletal Injury in an Infant and Child

A leading cause of death in children is accidents such as motor vehicle accidents, drowning, ingestions, and falls. Large amounts of resources are spent to both educate and prevent such accidents.

FRACTURES

In contrast to adults, when a child sustains an injury to an extremity, there is more often a fracture than ligamentous disruption because the ligaments are stronger than the bones. In general, fractures are less common than in adults. The bones of a child can withstand more bending stresses before breaking than adult bones. When fractures do occur, those involving the metaphysis and diaphysis can range from subtle (Fig. 29–1) to conspicuous. Metaphyseal and diaphyseal fractures range from bowing deformities, which is a number of microfractures along the concave edge resulting in a bowed configuration; to macrofractures involving the concave cortex, called "torus" fractures (Fig. 29–2); to fractures through the convex cortex, the so-called greenstick fracture; to complete through and through fractures.

In both the forearm and leg the bones are connected together by an interosseous membrane. When one of the bones of the pair is foreshortened for any reason, usually a fracture, something must happen to the other bone. In the forearm the fractures have characteristic appearances. A displaced or angulated fracture of the proximal ulna is usually associated with radial head dislocation (Monteggia fracture) (Fig. 29–3). A fracture of the distal radial shaft is associated with distal ulnar dislocation (Galeazzi fracture).

As with all of radiology, to evaluate a fracture, two views at right angles to each other are necessary (i.e., frontal and lateral). Routine views of the contralateral extremity should be avoided since it is usually unnecessary, costly, and involves excess radiation to the uninvolved area. If there is a question on one view, then possibly the contralateral side should be obtained in that one view only. An exception to this is whenever the hip is in question. In this instance, a view of the entire pelvis should be obtained in order to compare with the other side.

Salter-Harris Classification

When fractures involve the epiphyseal ends of the bones in growing children, growth plates are involved. This is because the ligaments and joint capsule are much stronger than the physis. Salter and Harris classify injuries to the physis and adjacent epiphysis and metaphysis into five traditional categories.

Type 1 involves only the physis. The radiographic appearance of these fractures is often minimal if the fracture is not displaced. Sometimes there is physeal widening, but more often there is only soft-tissue swelling with the apex of the swelling immediately over the physis. Type 2 injuries, which comprise approximately 75 percent

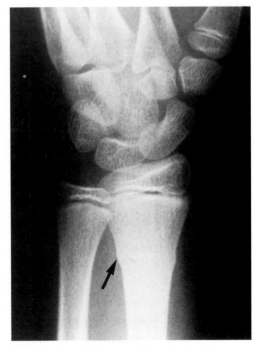

Figure 29–1. Subtle fracture of the distal radial metaphysis (arrow).

177

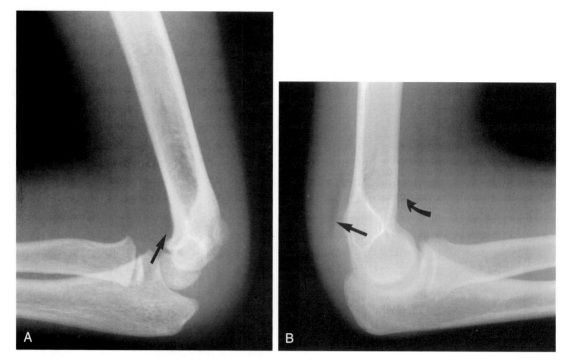

Figure 29–6. A, Normal lateral elbow showing a normal anterior fat pad *(arrow)* and no posterior fat pad. **B,** Elbow joint effusion with visualization of the posterior fat pad *(straight arrow)* and anterior elevation of the anterior fat pad *(curved arrow).*

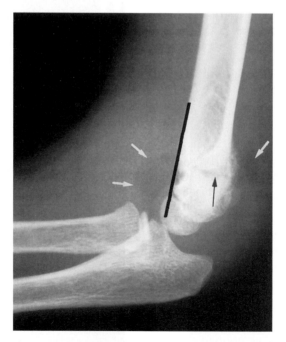

Figure 29–7. Supracondylar fracture of the distal humerus *(black arrow)* with a joint effusion *(white arrows).* Also note that the anterior humeral line does not pass through the anterior two thirds of the capitellar ossification center.

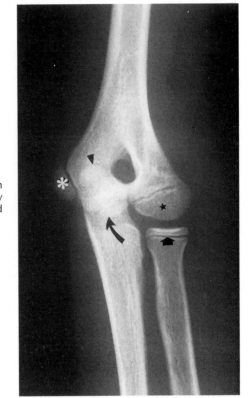

Figure 29–8. Normal ossification centers in the elbow: olecranon epiphysis *(arrowhead)*, capitellar epiphysis *(star)*, trochlea (frequently fragmented) *(curved arrow)*, medial epicondyle *(asterisk)*, radial head ossification *(broad arrow)*.

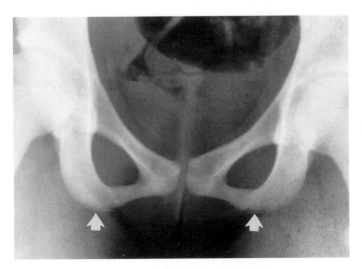

Figure 29–9. Ischial tuberosity apophyses *(arrows)* that can be pulled off while jumping hurdles.

pracondylar fracture can be diagnosed by drawing a line parallel to the anterior distal humeral shaft. Normally this line intersects the anterior two thirds of the capitellum. With a supracondylar fracture, the distal fracture fragment, including the capitellar ossification center, is posteriorly angulated. In this case, the anterior humeral line passes more anteriorly than normally. Adolescents tend to fracture the proximal radius. To exclude radial head dislocation, the radial head should line up with the capitellum in all projections. Other fractures tend to involve the epiphyses of the elbow. Therefore, it is important to know when to expect visualization of the epiphyses in the event that there is a displaced epiphyseal injury, making diagnosis of epiphyseal injury difficult. The order of epiphyseal appearance follows the mnemonic CRITOL: C = capitellum, R = radial head, I = internal or medial epicondyle, T = trochlea, O = olecranon, L = lateral epicondyle. Roughly, these epiphyses appear at 1, 3, 5, 7, 9, and 11 years of age (Fig 29–8).

Apophyseal Injuries

Apophyseal injuries can occur in the adolescent. An apophysis does not contribute to the longitudinal growth of the bone. These injuries are commonly seen in the pelvis (Fig. 29–9). A typical apophyseal injury occurs when the ischial tuberosity apophysis is pulled off during an activity such as jumping hurdles or performing the splits.

Another apophyseal injury occurs at the base of the fifth metatarsal. The normal apophysis can mimic a fracture. The growth plate for the apophysis is parallel to the long axis of the metatarsal. Fractures of the fifth metatarsal are seen as lucencies that are perpendicular to the long axis of the metatarsal (Fig. 29–10). When the growth plate appears widened with soft-tissue swelling over the area, then an apophyseal injury should be suspected.

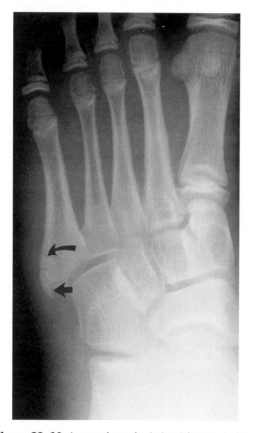

Figure 29–10. A normal apophysis *(straight arrow)* of the fifth metatarsal with a fracture of the same area *(curved arrow)*.

Chapter 30

Child Abuse

Child abuse has many names such as nonaccidental trauma, trauma X, battered child syndrome, shaken infant syndrome, and SCAN (suspected child abuse and neglect). Unfortunately, child abuse is commonly dealt with by pediatricians and pediatric radiologists alike. It occurs in all socioeconomic groups and races. If the diagnosis is missed, the child has a high risk of being severely beaten or killed the next time. Radiographically, skeletal and brain injuries are seen most frequently in patients under 2 years of age. These injuries are much less common in patients who are 4 years or older.

SHAKEN INFANT SYNDROME

Shaken infant syndrome is a specific type of abuse. In this syndrome the infants are shaken so violently that they suffer severe intracranial injury. The explanation for the intracranial injury is that the head in these infants makes up at least one quarter to one third of the total weight of the infant. When the infant is shaken, the head is extremely vulnerable to severe torque forces, which cause the bridging veins between the sagittal sinus and the dura to be sheared off, resulting in intracranial bleeding. These infants are frequently slammed against a hard object, which also causes severe intracranial injury as well as injuries to the rest of the skeleton. Because of the squeezing of the chest at the time of shaking, additional injuries occur. These injuries are rib fractures, lateral and posterior, as well as compression vertebral body fractures.

IMAGING IN CHILD ABUSE

Fractures are imaged with the skeletal survey or nuclear medicine bone scan or both. Brain parenchymal injuries are imaged with CT scans. The skeletal survey is a radiograph of every bone in the body in at least one projection. A routine skeletal survey includes three views of the skull (frontal, lateral, and Towne [to look at the lambdoidal suture]), frontal and lateral views of the trunk, and frontal views of the extremities to include the hands and feet.

The nuclear medicine bone scan is a procedure performed by intravenous injection of a radiopharmaceutical into the patient, and images are obtained approximately 3 hours after injection. The infant frequently needs to be sedated. The bone scan is more sensitive for bone pathology, but it is not specific. When compared with the cost of the skeletal survey, the cost of the bone scan is prohibitive as a first-line imaging modality. In addition, the patient receives more radiation with the bone scan. Therefore, the bone scan is used in those patients whose skeletal survey results are questionably positive or are negative but clinically highly suggest abuse or in those patients in whom old injuries are suspected that can no longer be seen on plain radiographs but in whom increased activity would be seen on bone scan. CT scanning of the brain should be done in addition to the skeletal survey in those infants who are less than 1 year of age or whose neurolgic examination results indicate an abnormality.

SKELETAL INJURIES SEEN WITH CHILD ABUSE

The hallmark of child abuse in the skeleton is multiple fractures in various stages of healing (Fig. 30–1). However, this hallmark is less commonly seen than is a single fracture. Other clues to the diagnosis of child abuse are fractures that are unusual for that particular child's age or are unusual in general. The "classic" fracture associated with child abuse is the corner metaphyseal fracture. This fracture results when the metaphysis is pulled off. If the fracture is viewed in tangent, it appears as a corner, but when seen *en face,* the entire metaphysis can be seen to be pulled off—the "bucket handle" fracture (Fig. 30–2). Therefore, the corner metaphyseal and bucket handle fracture are the same fracture viewed in two different ways. When this fracture is present, the diagnosis of abuse is virtually assured. However, it is seen much less commonly than the single fracture. The single fracture is usually present in the long bones (i.e., femur, tibia, humerus, radius, or ulna) (Fig. 30–3). The fracture is either spiral, implying a twisting mechanism, or trans-

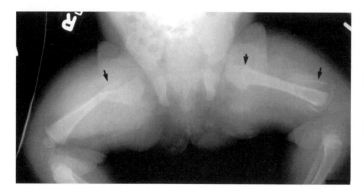

Figure 30–1. Multiple fractures in varying stages of healing are demonstrated in the lower extremities of this 2-month-old. Arrows denote the fractures. Those of the proximal femurs are more recent in age than is the fracture involving the distal left femur.

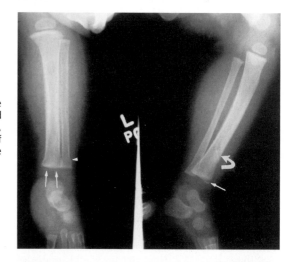

Figure 30–2. Straight arrows show the typical appearance of the corner metaphyseal fracture seen on the lateral and the "bucket handle" fracture seen on the frontal view. Also, the patient had a healing spiral fracture *(curved arrow)* of the distal tibia and an impaction fracture *(arrowhead)* of the distal fibula.

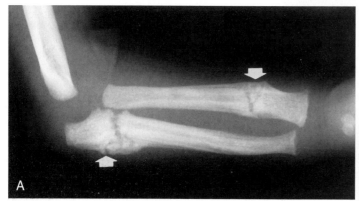

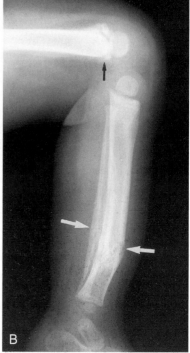

Figure 30–3. A, Forearm of infant with healing transverse fractures of radius and ulna *(arrows)*. **B,** Metaphyseal fracture of distal femur *(black arrow)* and healing fractures of distal tibia and fibula *(white arrows)*.

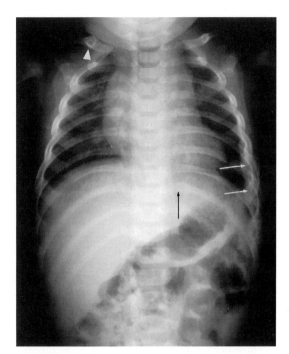

Figure 30–4. Healing rib fractures located in the typical position seen with squeezing the chest at the time of shaking—namely, laterally and posteriorly *(arrows)*. Also seen is a healing right clavicle fracture *(arrowhead)*.

verse, implying that a direct blow has occurred. The most commonly affected long bone is the femur followed by the tibia, which is usually asymptomatic and picked up on the skeletal survey and then followed by the humerus. (Obstetric injury is most commonly seen in the clavicle, followed by the humerus, and then by the femur.)

Unusual Fractures

Rib fractures are examples of unusual fractures (Fig. 30–4) because an infant's thoracic cage is elastic, resulting in few rib fractures even in major motor vehicle accidents. Also, unlike adults, rib fractures do not occur with cardiopulmonary resuscitation. Other unusual fractures include:

- Compression vertebral body fractures
- Scapular fractures
- Metacarpal and metatarsal fractures (accidental injuries to the hands and feet involve the phalanges)
- Bilateral clavicle fractures (usually accidental and obstetrical fractures are single)
- Corner metaphyseal fractures, which do not occur in the accidental setting in a patient with normal mineralization
- Transverse long bone fracture, which implies that the child could not have sustained it by him or herself

- Spiral fractures in the long bones of the infant who is not yet upright

A word of warning is needed here: **Beware of making the diagnosis of child abuse in the toddler.** Toddlers are capable of crawling and climbing and subsequently falling. Fractures can be sustained accidentally. These fractures frequently are not witnessed and usually involve the long bones, especially of the lower extremity. The "toddler's fracture" is a spiral fracture of the distal tibia (Fig. 30–5). It frequently is seen in those infants who are just beginning to walk. Despite the spiral nature of the fracture, it is an accidental injury and should not be mistaken for child abuse. Unusual fractures and the physical examination should help to diagnose child abuse in these patients.

Assessment of Bone Mineralization

Whenever the bones are being evaluated for possible abuse, an assessment of the mineralization of the bones must be made to exclude any predisposition to fracture such as that occurring in osteogenesis imperfecta. If the patient suffers from this condition at the age range being discussed with abuse, there is almost always osteopenia present, that is, the bones are too lucent (Fig. 30–6). Clinically, these patients often have abnormal dentition and blue sclera. Therefore an evaluation of child abuse in an infant should also in-

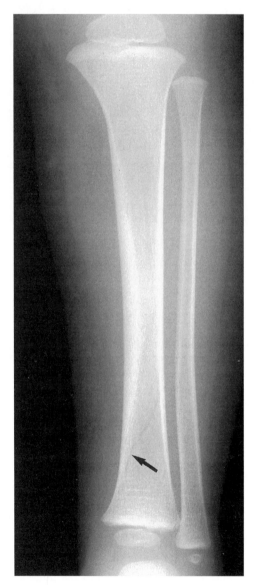

Figure 30–5. Frontal view showing spiral fracture of the distal tibia *(arrow)* (i.e., toddler's fracture).

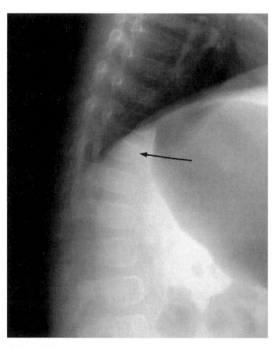

Figure 30–6. Lateral view of the thoracolumbar junction that demonstrates diffuse osteopenia of the bones and a slight compression fracture of a lower thoracic vertebral body *(arrow)* in this patient with osteogenesis imperfecta.

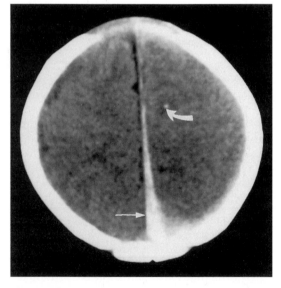

Figure 30–7. Classic interhemispheric subdural hematoma with high attenuation blood layering on one side of the falx *(straight arrow)*. Also present is a punctate hemorrhagic contusion *(curved arrow)*.

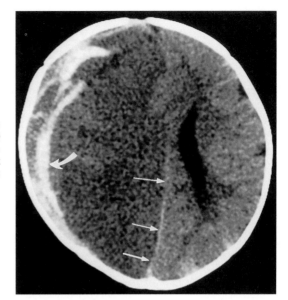

Figure 30–8. Diffuse cerebral edema is seen on the patient's right with shift of the midline to the left *(straight arrows)* and effacement of the right lateral ventricle. The mixed attenuation (high and intermediate) subdural blood is seen out laterally *(curved arrows)*, presumably indicating different ages of bleeding in this shaken infant.

volve a dysmorphologist just to exclude this rare condition, because it is always mentioned in the courtroom as a possibility to explain the injuries sustained.

ABNORMAL HEAD CT SCAN IN THE ABUSED CHILD

An interhemispheric subdural hematoma is a characteristic of shaken infant syndrome and is seen as an abnormality on a CT scan. This blood results from the disruption of the bridging cerebral veins between the dura and sagittal sinus. Radiographically, this is seen as an eccentric crescent of high attenuation layering posteriorly up against the falx in the interhemispheric fissure (Fig. 30–7). The finding of an interhemispheric subdural is nearly pathognomic of shaken infant syndrome. Other much less specific findings on head CT include cerebral edema (Fig. 30–8),

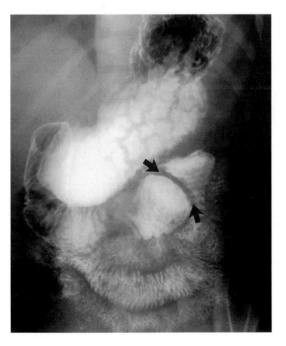

Figure 30–9. Upper gastrointestinal examination showing dilated duodenum at the duodenal-jejunal junction. The persistent lucency *(arrows)* distal to the dilation represented an adhesion from an old duodenal perforation.

hemorrhagic contusions, and skull fracture. (Note: Accidental brain injury in an infant is rare in the absence of a major motor vehicle accident.)

SOFT-TISSUE INJURIES OF THE ABUSED CHILD

Other injuries that can result from child abuse are soft-tissue injuries. Pancreatitis in a child is caused by trauma in one third of all cases. Some of the trauma is from nonaccidental injury. Ruptured viscus from a direct blow to the abdomen usually involves the small bowel where it crosses the spine. Less severe injury involves the duodenum and results in a duodenal hematoma. The hematoma may be large enough to cause obstruction with resultant vomiting. Any abused child that starts to vomit may have a bowel injury, which should be evaluated by UGI (Fig. 30–9).

Chapter 31

The Limping Toddler

The limping child typically presents in the toddler age range. These children cannot really tell the examiner where it hurts. The main differential causes of this problem include the "toddler's fracture," septic hip, and discitis. Other less common causes include osteomyelitis and occult malignancy. Therefore the radiographic evaluation of this complaint should include visualization of the lumbar spine down to the foot. If the radiographs are normal, nuclear medicine bone scanning may need to be performed to evaluate for the occult injury.

TODDLER'S FRACTURE

The toddler's fracture originally was described as a spiral fracture seen in the tibia in this age group. It was typically seen in toddlers who were just beginning to walk. They would plant their tennis-shoed foot down and turn to walk away, but the foot would not go with their bodies. This mechanism would result in a twisting force that would subsequently cause the spiral-type fracture (Fig. 31–1). Most of the time the event would be unwitnessed. Note: This fracture should not be considered a result of child abuse. Now, the toddler's fracture is also described as a stress-type fracture and can involve both the calcaneus and the cuboid (Fig. 31–2). Both of these latter injuries are usually only picked up on bone scanning initially. When they start to heal with sclerosis, they can then be appreciated on the plain radiographs.

DISCITIS

Discitis typically occurs in the toddler age group but there is another peak in early adolescence. The infection typically starts in the disc in children and then spreads to the adjoining verte-

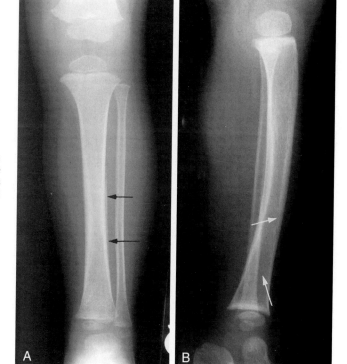

Figure 31–1. A, Healing toddler's fracture with periosteal new bone seen laterally *(arrows).* The fracture itself is difficult to see. **B,** The toddler's fracture can better be appreciated on the lateral view *(arrows).*

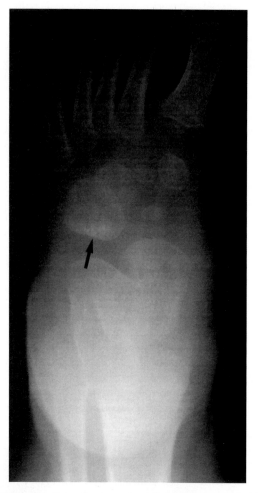

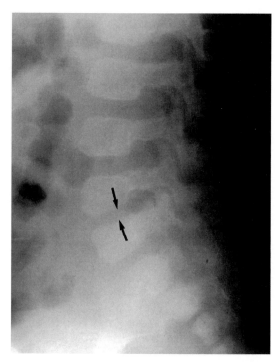

Figure 31–3. Lateral view showing discitis with narrowing of the L4-5 disc space *(arrows)*. In addition, there is poor definition of the vertebral body endplates due to inflammation.

Figure 31–2. Another type of toddler's fracture is a cuboid injury that is thought to result from either jumping off a high position or to represent a stress-type or overuse fracture. The proximal cuboid is sclerotic *(arrow)* in comparison with the remaining bones of the foot, which indicates healing.

bral body endplates. Causal agents can be found approximately 50 percent of the time and most commonly involve *Staphylococcus aureus.*

Radiographically, the process is most commonly seen in the L3-4 to L4-5 disc spaces (Fig. 31–3). On a normal lateral view the disc spaces get larger as one proceeds inferiorly, except at L5-S1. With discitis, this rule is broken, and the involved disc space is narrower than the one above. However, this finding is not seen typically until at least 2 to 4 weeks after symptoms appear. Bone scanning and MRI can pick up the abnormality early in the course of the disease.

On bone scan the vertebral bodies above and below the affected disc show increased uptake because the process has spread from the disc to the adjacent endplates (Fig. 31–4). MRI likewise

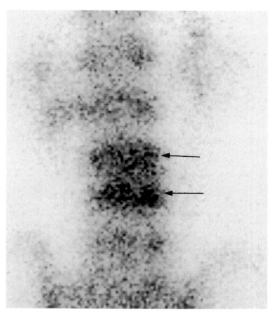

Figure 31–4. Bone scan image of lumbar spine in a patient with discitis at the L3-4 level. Increased activity *(arrows)* of the vertebral bodies is seen above and below the involved disc.

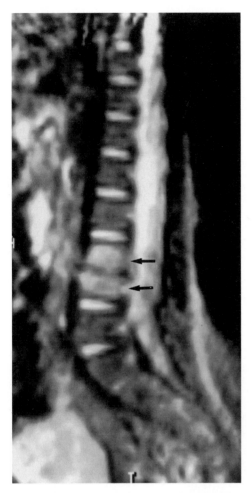

Figure 31–5. MRI confirming the L3-4 discitis with increased signal intensity of the involved vertebral bodies *(arrows)* on T2-weighted images.

shows increased signal on T2-weighted images in the adjacent vertebral bodies (Fig. 31–5). As time goes on, the plain films show not only loss of disc space height but also sclerosis of the adjacent endplates.

SEPTIC HIP

Septic hip is a surgical emergency in that any time there is a joint effusion in the hip, vascularity is compromised by the increased pressure. If the pressure is not relieved, the femoral head could become infarcted. The initial plain films may show a joint effusion, which is diagnosed by comparing the uninvolved side to the affected one. Note: If the hip needs to be radiographed, the pelvis should be filmed. The distance between the femoral metaphysis and the acetabulum (this landmark looks like a teardrop) should be less

than 2 millimeters from side to side (Fig. 31–6). If greater than this, a joint effusion should be suspected. The joint should be tapped immediately to relieve pressure. If the plain films are negative, imaging of the joint with ultrasound can be obtained or a nuclear medicine bone scan can be done. The latter can evaluate possible vascular compromise by showing a "cold" femoral head. Ultrasound can reveal the joint effusion, especially when compared with the normal side (Fig. 31–7). On ultrasound, the configuration of the soft tissue planes adjacent to the femoral shaft confirms the diagnosis of effusion rather than the absolute measurement of the planes. With a hip effusion, the planes of the joint capsule are convex relative to the concavity of the femoral metaphysis. With no joint effusion these planes are concave and parallel to the femoral metaphysis. This examination for hip effusion can be performed on a patient of any age. Large body habitus is the only limiting factor.

OSTEOMYELITIS

The most common organism to cause osteomyelitis is *Staphylococcus aureus*. The earliest radio-

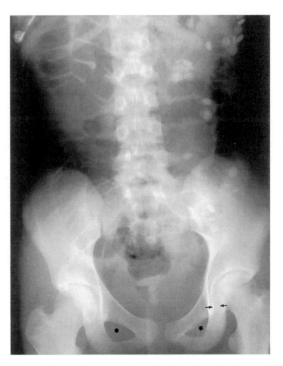

Figure 31–6. The arrows show the "teardrop" to femoral head distance *(arrows)*. To compare with the other side accurately, the pelvis needs to be straight. In this patient there is obliquity of the pelvis as seen by the asymmetry of the pubic rings *(asterisks)*. Incidental note is made of iron tablets in the intestine.

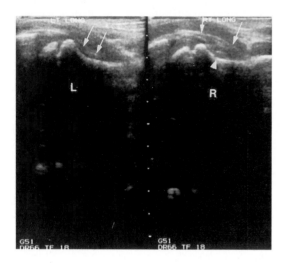

Figure 31–7. Ultrasound imaging of right hip joint effusion where the planes of the joint capsule echoes are convex *(arrows)* compared to the metaphysis of the femoral shaft *(arrowhead)*. The left normal side shows the planes concave *(arrows)*.

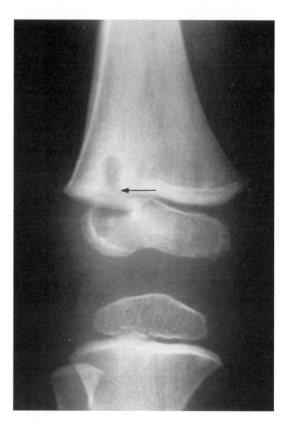

Figure 31–8. Lytic area in the distal femoral metaphysis *(arrow)* is due to osteomyelitis.

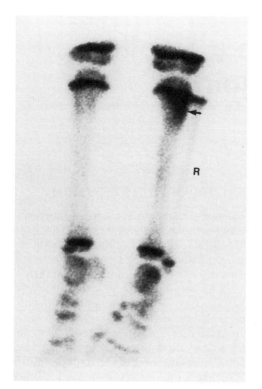

Figure 31–9. Nuclear medicine bone scan shows increased activity in the right proximal tibia in this posterior image. The flame-shaped *(arrow)* area of the increased metaphyseal activity is characteristic.

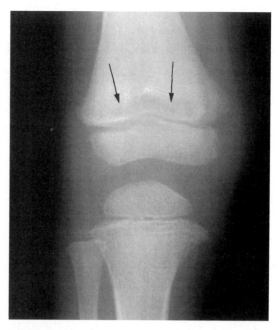

Figure 31–10. Metaphyseal lucencies *(arrows)* in this leukemia patient.

graphic findings are soft-tissue swelling followed by bone erosion, which occurs several days into the infection (Fig. 31–8). Bone scan shows increased activity earlier than the plain films show lytic areas (Fig. 31–9). This increased activity is characteristically flame-shaped, extending away from the normally "hot" physis.

MALIGNANCY

The most common malignancy to result in leg pain in a child is leukemia. The radiographs may be a clue to the underlying problem if they show either diffuse osteopenia or metaphyseal lucency (Fig. 31–10). Normally the metaphysis of a long bone is sclerotic. When leukemia or neuroblastoma is present, this sclerosis is replaced by lucency. The differential diagnosis of these lucencies includes disuse and systemic steroids.

Chapter 32

The Child with a Swollen Joint or Joints

In this chapter the differential diagnosis mainly includes septic joint (both acute bacterial and chronic granulomatous), hemophiliac arthropathy, and juvenile chronic arthritis (i.e., juvenile rheumatoid arthritis). All the chronic causes of joint abnormalities have similar radiographic findings in that there is diffuse osteopenia and overgrowth of the epiphyses, both of which are due to the chronic hyperemia (Fig. 32–1). Usually a joint effusion is also present. In the acute septic joint, only the joint effusion is seen since the other findings previously mentioned are more chronic. If the process involves the adjacent bone (i.e., osteomyelitis), then bony erosions are seen as well (Fig. 32–2).

IMAGING OF JOINT EFFUSION

A joint effusion in the knee is diagnosed by looking in the space above the patella and anterior to the distal femur but just posterior to the suprapatellar tendon. This space should be relatively lucent since it usually contains fat. When there is an effusion, the lucency is replaced by water density, which is the same as the surrounding muscle. In the adolescent the water density can be measured in the anteroposterior direction. If it measures 10 millimeters, a joint effusion is definitely present (Fig. 32–3). If the measurement is less than 6 millimeters, there is no effusion. If

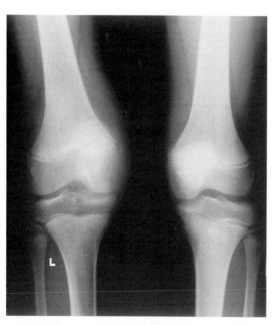

Figure 32–1. Frontal view of both knees showing osteopenia on the left compared to the normal right knee. The epiphyses on the osteopenic side are larger than those on the right in this patient with juvenile rheumatoid arthritis.

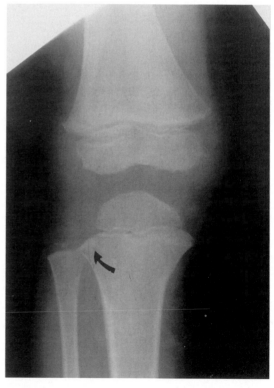

Figure 32–2. Subtle area of lucency *(arrow)* that represented acute osteomyelitis.

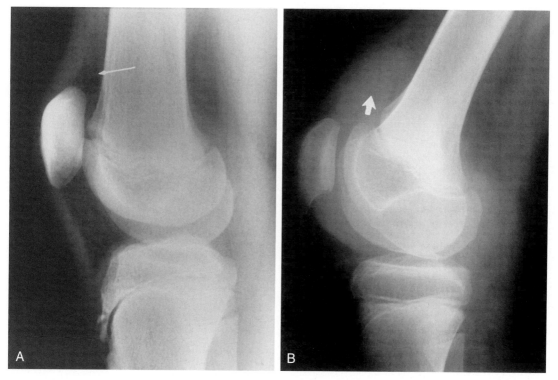

Figure 32–3. A, Normal lateral view of knee with fat *(arrow)* seen in the space anterior to the distal femur. **B,** Knee joint effusion with the suprapatellar fat obliterated *(arrow).*

the water density is between 6 and 9 millimeters, an effusion may be present. In the more immature knee the detection of a joint effusion can be more difficult. The easiest way to diagnose one is to see obscuration of the cartilaginous portions of the epiphyses about the knee, which normally are outlined by fat.

A joint effusion in the ankle can be difficult to diagnose, but there is a radiolucent triangle just anterior to the ankle joint that becomes obliterated when there is an effusion (Fig. 32–4). Likewise there is a similar finding just posterior to the ankle joint. The anterior portion is more sensitive and specific for effusion, since the posterior aspect can be simulated by plantar flexion of the foot. A joint effusion in the elbow, as discussed in Chapter 29, causes displacement of the fat pads (Fig. 29–6). Likewise, diagnosis of a hip effusion is also discussed in Chapter 31 (Fig. 31–7).

HEMOPHILIC ARTHROPATHY

Hemophilic arthropathy tends to involve the large joints—knees, elbows, and ankles—but in an asymmetric fashion. Because of the repetitive bleeding that occurs in these patients, the epiphyses not only become overgrown but also have

well-defined erosions (Fig. 32–5). In addition, the soft tissues about the affected joint in hemophilia are denser than usual because of the chronic bloody effusions. The density is due to the presence of hemosiderin deposition in the tissues.

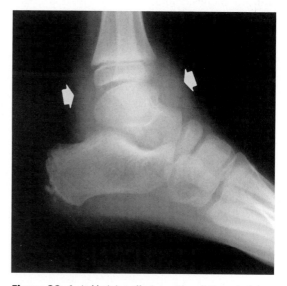

Figure 32–4. Ankle joint effusion with soft tissue bulging anterior and posterior to the joint *(arrows).*

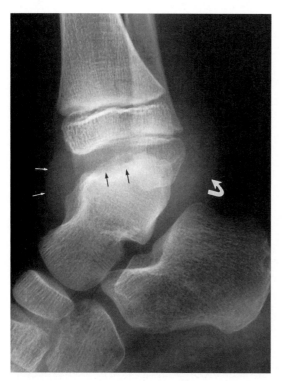

Figure 32–5. Ankle joint effusion with obliteration of the fat anterior *(white arrows)* and posterior *(curved arrow)*. There is bone erosion of the talar done *(black arrows)* due to hemophilic arthropathy.

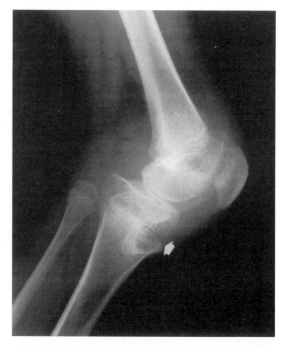

Figure 32–6. Tuberculous arthritis. The knee is diffusely osteopenic, and there is bony erosion in the proximal anterior tibia *(arrow)*.

JUVENILE RHEUMATOID ARTHRITIS

Juvenile rheumatoid arthritis (JRA) affects the large joints, as does hemophilia, before the small joints of the hands and feet are affected. This entity is more common in girls. There is overgrowth of the epiphyses due to hyperemia. Juxtaarticular osteoporosis (Fig. 32–1) and erosions are present at ligamentous sites. Obviously, to differentiate this disorder from hemophilia, the clinical history should be obtained.

SEPTIC ARTHRITIS

In acute septic arthritis, joint destruction is seen early in the course of the infection. However, with the more indolent infectious processes, such as tuberculosis or fungal infections, the radiographic findings are similar to those discussed with JRA and hemophilia. Specifically, with tuberculosis, the larger joints are again most commonly affected. There is osteopenia, frequently joint effusion particularly in the knee, and erosions along joint margins (Fig. 32–6).

Chapter 33

The Older Child or Adolescent with Lower Extremity Pain

The differential diagnosis of patients with this symptom includes trauma (occult and nonoccult); Legg-Calvé-Perthes disease; slipped capital femoral epiphysis; bone tumors, both benign and malignant; infection or inflammation; and some congenital conditions.

TRAUMA

With occult trauma (i.e., stress fractures), radiographs are usually normal in the acute period. In approximately 10 to 14 days, healing periosteal new bone is usually seen, which helps to confirm the diagnosis. Nuclear medicine bone scanning is much more sensitive than plain films, and the study is positive much earlier than the radiographs. In the imaging of potential stress fractures, if the initial films are negative, either a bone scan should be obtained immediately or if the diagnosis does not need to be made immediately, more plain radiographs should be done in approximately 2 weeks. MRI can also be performed instead of nuclear medicine, although it is more expensive. Abnormal signal in the marrow is seen with stress fractures.

Typical places for stress fractures are the 3rd and 4th metatarsals. (This is known as the "march fracture," because it is frequent in new military recruits.) Another common location is the proximal tibia. When it occurs in this location, it is seen posteriorly along the proximal tibial diaphysis (Fig. 33–1). Femoral neck stress fractures are also seen on occasion, as well as along the femoral diaphysis (Fig. 33–2).

Nonoccult trauma should be evaluated by plain radiographs first. As in all radiology, views at right angles to one another should be obtained. If the fracture involves the pelvis, CT of the pelvis should also be obtained. Fractures of the acetabulum are much better evaluated by CT. Sometimes three-dimensional reconstruction of the fracture can be obtained on a computer. However, the three-dimensional reconstruction requires obtaining thin slices consecutively through the area of interest, which increases radiation to the patient. The computer then reconstructs the images in any plane desired.

As opposed to patients who can experience pain with trauma, patients who have no sensation to trauma in an area have joints that can have a distinctive radiographic appearance. Patients who can feel fractures usually stop using the area, which results in disuse. The fracture usually heals, and then the mineralization returns to near normal. Insensate patients continue to use the injured part because of the lack of feeling. As a result, the joint frequently becomes extremely disorganized with multiple fracture fragments and maintenance

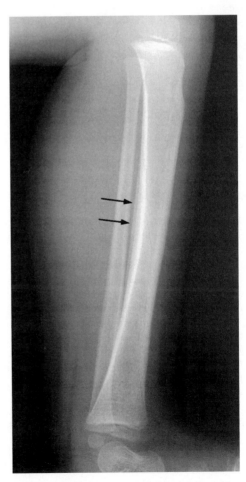

Figure 33–1. Healing toddler's fracture (a type of stress fracture) as demonstrated by periosteal new bone seen along the posterior tibia *(arrows)*.

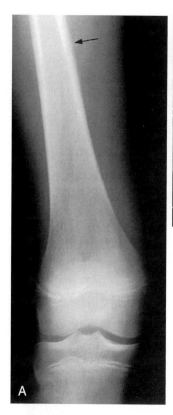

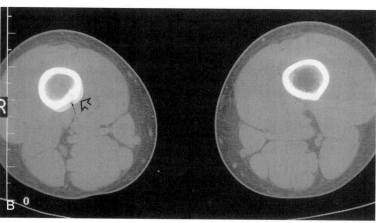

Figure 33–2. A, Femoral shaft shows stress fracture demonstrated by subtle periosteal new bone *(arrow).* **B,** CT of same patient showing fracture of the cortex *(straight arrow)* surrounded by periosteal new bone *(open arrow).*

of sclerosis. The term for this appearance is Charcot arthropathy (Fig. 33–3).

LEGG-CALVÉ-PERTHES DISEASE

Legg-Calvé-Perthes (LCP) disease is idiopathic osteonecrosis of the femoral head. It is more commonly seen in boys in the age range of 4 to 11 years with a peak at 6 years. The condition can be bilateral 10 percent of the time, but the radiographic findings, as discussed below, are never symmetric. The process occurs in a sequential, not simultaneous, fashion. If the radiographic changes are bilaterally symmetric, the osteonecrosis is no longer idiopathic and most likely is due to some underlying condition such as sickle cell disease or Gaucher disease.

By the time the patient seeks medical attention, the pain has usually existed for several weeks. Pelvic radiographs, in both frontal and frog-leg lateral views, are the most commonly used imaging modality to make this diagnosis. Again, comparison with the opposite and presumed asymptomatic hip is essential. However, the plain films can be normal. In these cases other imaging modalities can be obtained, such as MRI or nu-

clear medicine bone scan. MRI can show an area of decreased signal intensity in the femoral head long before the femoral head changes can be seen radiographically. The decreased signal is due to devascularization. Nuclear medicine bone scanning can show decreased perfusion on the radionuclide angiogram phase and then a "cold" head on the delayed phase of the bone scan.

Plain Film Findings

The first radiographic finding in the early phases of the disease is osteopenia from disuse. Next is apparent joint space widening from soft-tissue edema. Then there is a subchondral fracture—the "crescent sign" seen just under the edge of the epiphysis (Fig. 33–4). The femoral head then becomes diffusely sclerotic and loses height and fragments. This is the dissolution phase. Eventually the head remineralizes with deformity, depending on how much of the femoral head was initially involved. If there was total head involvement, the femoral head takes on a "mushroom" appearance (Fig. 33–5). In the initial phase of the disease, the patients are frequently treated in an abduction brace. This is thought to keep the

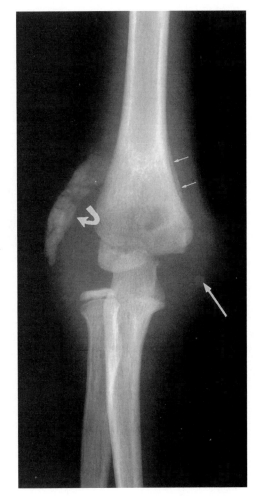

Figure 33–3. Charcot elbow joint. The mineralization is normal. There is a healing fracture of the distal humerus *(small arrows)*, a displaced medial epicondyle fracture *(large straight arrow)*, joint dislocation—the ulna and radius are displaced laterally from the humerus—and an ossifying hematoma (myositis) in the soft tissues *(curved arrow)*.

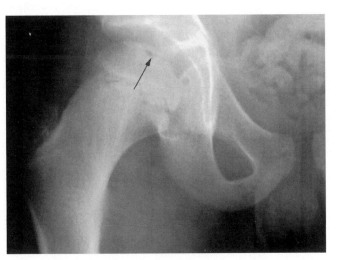

Figure 33–4. Legg-Calvé-Perthes (idiopathic osteonecrosis) with subchondral lucency *(arrow)*.

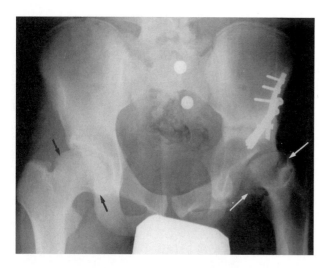

Figure 33–5. Patient with previous bilateral osteonecrosis and resultant mushroom deformities *(arrows)*. An osteotomy of the left acetabulum has been performed to make for better femoral head coverage.

femoral heads directed more toward the acetabulum in the hope of attaining more concentric remineralization of the femoral head and acetabulum. Legg-Calvé-Perthes, as stated earlier, is idiopathic osteonecrosis. There are underlying conditions that can cause osteonecrosis such as the following: systemic steroids (the femoral heads can be symmetrically affected), septic hip, some marrow replacement disorder such as Gaucher disease, and developmental dysplasia of the hip (Fig. 33–6). In the latter condition the osteonecrosis usually occurs at an earlier age than LCP and the acetabulum is more dysplastic.

SLIPPED CAPITAL FEMORAL EPIPHYSIS

Typically, at the onset of the adolescent growth spurt, slipped capital femoral epiphysis (SCFE) can occur. This condition occurs more frequently in males and is bilateral in about 10 percent of cases. The patients are usually obese, which probably results in abnormal stresses on the proximal femoral physis. Therefore, SCFE may be a stress fracture. It is also similar to a Salter-Harris type 1 fracture. There is a risk of osteonecrosis of the femoral head in this condition. Growth hormone

Figure 33–6. Osteonecrosis secondary to developmental dysplasia of the hip. The typical changes of osteonecrosis are seen with flattening and sclerosis of the femoral head *(arrow)*. Usually the osteonecrosis changes occur earlier than the typical age range of LCP.

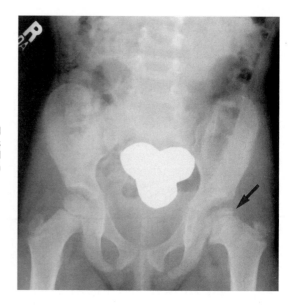

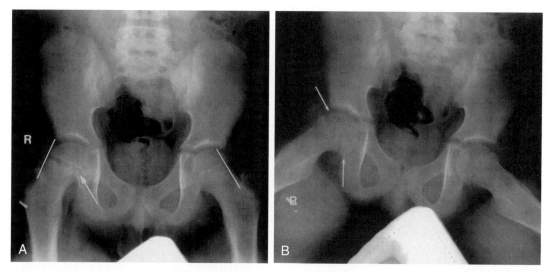

Figure 33–7. A, Frontal view of patient with slipped capital femoral epiphysis (SCFE) on the right. The physis is wider on the right than the left *(arrow)*, and a line drawn along the lateral femoral neck on this side does not intersect the femoral head as it does on the left. **B,** The typical appearance of the "ice cream scoop falling off the cone" in SCFE on the right *(arrows)*.

therapy can be associated with SCFE. Therefore, all patients about to start this therapy need a screening pelvis radiograph. There may be an association of hypothyroidism associated with SCFE, but this theory is controversial.

When the diagnosis is made, the treatment involves iatrogenic fusion of the physis. Physeal fusion prevents further slippage, thereby decreasing the risk of vascular compromise to the femoral head with subsequent osteonecrosis. The surgery for this condition is to pin the femoral neck through the physis and into the femoral head without changing the alignment of the original deformity; that is, the hip is pinned in deformity. The reason for pinning in deformity is to try to reduce the incidence of osteonecrosis that might occur if the fracture were reduced.

Radiographic Findings

Diagnosis of SCFE is made by plain pelvis radiographs in both the frontal and frog-leg position. Obtaining the frog-leg view is controversial in this diagnosis. Some believe that the slipping of the femoral head can be made worse by this position and that a cross-table lateral should be done instead. The detection of SCFE can be difficult on the frontal view. There may be a slight widening of the physis compared to the contralateral side (Fig. 33–7A). In addition, on the affected side a line drawn parallel to the outer aspect of the

femoral neck should barely intersect the femoral head normally. With SCFE, this line misses the head. On the frog-leg view, the diagnosis is usually readily apparent when compared with the normal side. If the femoral head-neck complex is compared to an ice cream cone, with the neck being the cone and the head being the scoop of ice cream, it looks as if the scoop of ice cream has fallen off the cone (Fig. 33–7B).

BONE TUMORS

In general, bone tumors are rare. The incidence of bone tumors is approximately 0.02 percent. The incidence of malignant bone tumors is only a small percentage of these at 0.0056 percent.

Radiographic Findings

Bone tumors are divided radiographically into benign and malignant by several different criteria. A benign lesion has extremely well defined borders so that the lesion can be separated from normal bone easily. This appearance is called geographic margination (Fig. 33–8). In addition, a benign lesion usually has a sclerotic rim around it. If there is periosteal new bone about the lesion, it is thickened and appears solid. A few of the more common benign bone lesions are simple cyst, fibrous cortical defect, aneurysmal bone cyst, and fibrous dysplasia. In malignant lesions, a

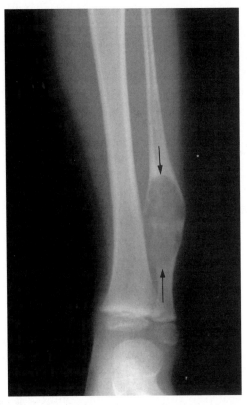

Figure 33–8. Benign bone lesion (fibrous dysplasia) as shown by the well-defined margins of this lesion *(arrows)*.

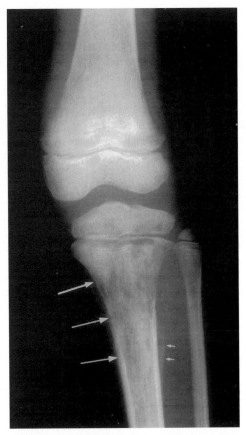

Figure 33–9. Patient with leukemic infiltration of bones demonstrating a permeative pattern of the abnormal bone *(large arrows)* compared to the normal. There is immature periosteal new bone seen, as well *(small arrows)*.

poorly defined edge of the lesion is seen when compared with normal bone. This appearance is called a poorly defined zone of transition (Fig. 33–9). The lesion frequently appears moth eaten. When there is periosteal new bone formation, it is thin and immature and can have a laminated or sunburst appearance. Some lesions are difficult to characterize by plain film, which makes biopsy absolutely necessary. Some more commonly seen malignant lesions are osteosarcoma, Ewing sarcoma, Langerhans cell histiocytosis, and bony metastases. (Note: Chronic osteomyelitis can simulate malignancy.)

Benign Bone Lesions

Simple Bone Cyst. A simple bone cyst, also known as a unicameral bone cyst, is most commonly seen in the proximal humerus but can be seen in the femoral neck. The lesion starts in the proximal metaphysis of the bone and is as wide as the metaphysis (Fig. 33–10). With growth of the long bone, the lesion appears to migrate down the shaft. The lesion maintains its original width and appears as a bulge of lucent bone in the diaphysis. These lesions usually present with a fracture through it (i.e., a pathological fracture). Since the cyst is fluid-filled, if there is a fracture through it, there may be a piece of bone seen that floats to the bottom of the cyst—the so-called "fallen fragment" sign. Treatment after fracture healing is to sclerose the cyst, usually with steroid injected into the cyst. After skeletal maturity is reached, the lesion usually heals and essentially disappears.

Fibrous Cortical Defect. Fibrous cortical defects, as the name implies, arise in the cortex of the bone in the metaphyseal region. They are usually oval and approximately 1 to 2 centimeters in length. They have a sclerotic margin and are most frequently seen about the knee (Fig. 33–11). They disappear in 2 to 4 years. Lesions larger than this that start to encroach on the medullary cavity are called nonossifying fibromas.

Aneurysmal Bone Cysts. Aneurysmal bone cysts are bubbly-like, expansile lesions that have a predilection for the posterior elements of the spine (as discussed in Chapter 33), the metaphyseal portion of the long bones, and the pelvis. The lesion is seen in adolescents primarily and contains blood-filled cystic spaces. The bony cortex is ballooned out by the lesion and is extremely thin and barely visible by plain film. Usually no periosteal bone is seen unless the lesion has fractured. On MRI and CT (Fig. 34–11) the lesion frequently shows fluid-fluid levels due to blood layering.

Fibrous Dysplasia. Fibrous dysplasia can be in one bone (monostotic) or in several bones (polyostotic). The single bone appearance will be discussed in this section. The lesions are seen in the metaphyseal portion of the long bones (Fig. 33–8). The classic description of the lesion is of "ground glass"—almost a radiolucent appearance with a well-defined border. Other common locations include the skull and pelvis.

Malignant Bone Lesions

Osteosarcoma. Osteosarcoma is most commonly seen in adolescents and is localized about the knee, although it can occur almost anywhere. The classic appearance is that of a lesion in the metaphyseal-diaphyseal region of the long bone with predominant sclerosis of the lesion, but there can be lucency as well. The lesion blends imperceptively with the surrounding normal bone. The lesion breaks out of the cortex producing immature periosteal new bone that looks like a sunburst (Fig. 33–12) or has a layered look (laminated). The lesion is first evaluated by plain film but then is usually imaged by both nuclear medicine bone scan and MRI. On bone scan the lesion is intensely hot because of the hypervascular nature of the

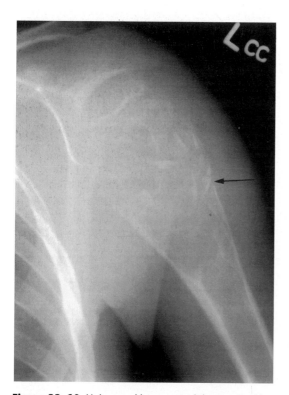

Figure 33–10. Unicameral bone cyst of the proximal humerus with a fracture through it (i.e., pathologic fracture) *(arrow)*.

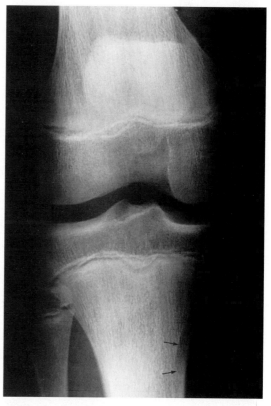

Figure 33–11. Fibrous cortical defect proximal medial tibial metaphysis *(arrows)*. The lesion is eccentric and cortically based. It has well-defined margins and usually disappears once skeletal maturity has been attained.

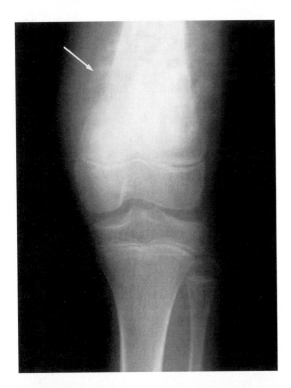

Figure 33–12. Typical osteosarcoma of the distal femoral metaphysis. The lesion is predominantly sclerotic with immature periosteal new bone *(arrow)* similar to a sunburst pattern.

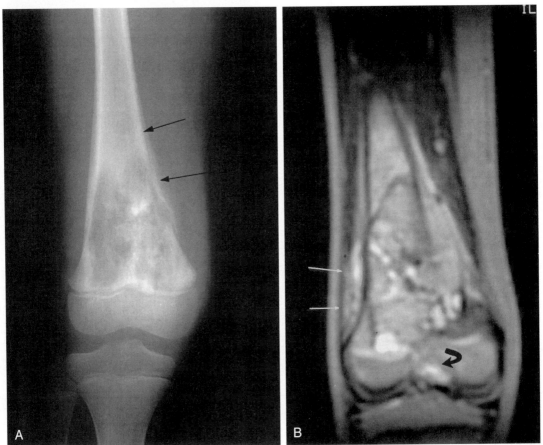

Figure 33–13. A, Predominantly lytic distal femoral osteosarcoma. The periosteal new bone is laminated in the lesion *(arrows).* **B,** MRI of the same lesion showing the soft-tissue component *(straight arrows)* as well as the epiphyseal extension *(curved arrow)* of the tumor not seen on plain film.

tumor. Osteosarcoma metastases are intensely hot as well. MRI accurately evaluates the soft-tissue component of the lesion, the extent of the medullary cavity involvement (Fig. 33–13), and skip lesions within the medullary cavity. These images are important when planning for limb-salvage procedures. When the lesion is predominantly lytic, the MRI may show fluid-fluid levels, indicating that the histologic type is that of the telangiectatic variety.

Since osteosarcomas typically metastasize to the lungs and other bones, imaging of the lungs is performed by both CT scan and plain film chest radiograph, as well as nuclear medicine bone scan. CT scan detects lung metastases earlier than chest radiograph. Bone scan detects bone metastases earlier than radiographs.

Ewing Sarcoma. Ewing sarcoma is also seen in adolescents and has a predilection for flat bone areas like the pelvis (Fig. 33–14) and ribs, as well as the long bones such as the femur. The lesion is more often diaphyseal than is osteosarcoma. It is characteristically lytic and elongated with laminated periosteal new bone. Imaging evaluation is similar to osteosarcoma with plain films of the affected bone, MRI, nuclear medicine bone scan, CT scan of the lungs, and plain chest radiographs. Bone scan of the lesion is not as hyperintense as osteosarcoma unless there is a pathologic fracture through the lesion.

Langerhans Cell Histiocytosis. Langerhans cell histiocytosis can be systemic or localized. When systemic, the process results in lytic bone lesions anywhere in the skeleton. There is frequently infiltration of the soft tissues. Infiltration of the soft tissues results in an interstitial lung pattern, organomegaly, diabetes insipidus (when the pituitary stalk is infiltrated), or draining ear (when the mastoids and inner ear are involved).

Radiographic Findings

Skeleton. The lytic lesions usually do not have a sclerotic rim until treated and can be in any portion of the bone. The calvarium is the most commonly involved portion of the skeleton (Fig. 33–15). In this location the edges of the lesion look beveled (Fig. 34–13) because the lesion arises in the diploic space and erodes the outer and inner tables of the skull at varying rates. Imaging of the bony lesions in this entity is with skeletal survey almost exclusively, because the nuclear medicine bone scan is usually normal unless there has been a fracture through these lesions.

Soft Tissues. MRI of the brain can help evaluate the mastoid area and pituitary stalk when symptoms suggest involvement in these regions. Ultrasound can be used to diagnose organomegaly in the abdomen, and plain chest radiographs can evaluate possible interstitial lung disease.

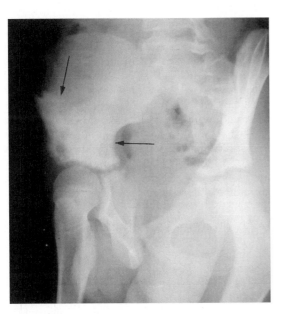

Figure 33–14. Ewing sarcoma of the right iliac bone with both lytic and sclerotic components *(arrows)*. The lesion blends imperceptively with the normal bone.

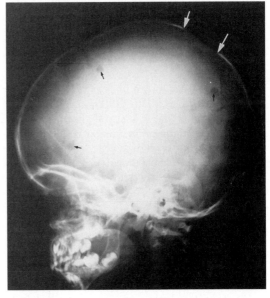

Figure 33–15. Histiocytosis involving the calvarium. Several small lytic lesions are seen *(black arrows)*, and one large lesion is seen in tangent *(white arrows)*.

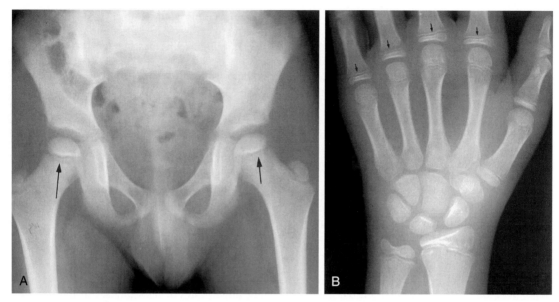

Figure 33–16. A, Metaphyseal lucencies in the proximal femoral metaphyses *(arrows)*. Normally, these areas are sclerotic. **B,** A similar appearance to the hand with metaphyseal lucencies seen best in the proximal phalangeal metaphyses *(arrows)*.

Metastases

Metastases to the skeleton in the pediatric age group are usually due to leukemia, neuroblastoma, rhabdomyosarcoma, or lymphoma. These entities are indistinguishable on plain film and need either biopsy or clinical data to determine their etiology. The lesions are characteristically lytic and need to be evaluated by skeletal survey, because they are difficult to see on nuclear medicine bone scan. The lesions can vary from frank destructive lesions, usually located in the metaphyseal regions of any of the bones, to metaphyseal lucent lines (Fig. 33–16) seen in a similar location. Metaphyseal lucent lines are not specific for these malignancies. In the differential of metaphyseal lucent lines there is also disuse osteopenia, systemic steroid ingestion, Langerhans cell histiocytosis, and sickle cell disease. Sometimes the skeleton is diffusely osteopenic (too lucent) without focal abnormality. This appearance can be seen with leukemia and in some hepatoblastoma patients.

MISCELLANEOUS

Infection

Acute bacterial infection causes lytic ill-defined lesions. More chronic bacterial infections are of-ten diffusely sclerotic, but the periosteal new bone seen is mature and thick (Fig. 33–17). Granulomatous infection causes more indolent changes such as diffuse osteopenia and, frequently, a well-defined lytic area (Fig. 33–18).

Inflammation or Arthritis

Sacroiliitis can be the first presentation of a systemic disorder, such as inflammatory bowel disease or rheumatic arthritides. Plain films of the sacroiliac joints can be difficult to evaluate and frequently need to be imaged by either nuclear medicine or CT scan (Fig. 33–19). Hemophiliac arthritis eventually results in bony erosions due to the hyperemic synovium. The bony changes are indistinguishable from granulomatous arthritides (Fig. 33–20). The large joints such as elbows, knees, and ankles are typically involved in an asymmetric fashion.

Congenital

Some congenital conditions such as undiagnosed developmental dysplasia of the hip (Fig. 33–21) can cause lower extremity pain. In neurologically impaired patients acquired dislocation can be due to the tight adductor muscles, which frequently are present. The acetabulum is much

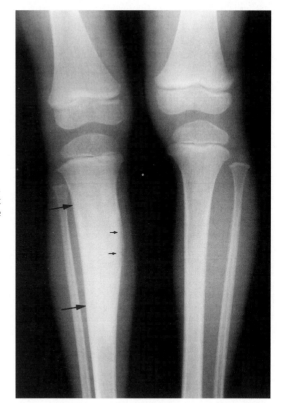

Figure 33–17. Chronic osteomyelitis with diffuse sclerosis, tibial shaft thickening and deformity *(large arrows)*. The lytic area was the site of a foreign body *(small arrows)* that gave rise to the osteomyelitis.

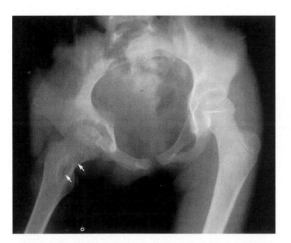

Figure 33–18. Tuberculosis infection with diffuse osteopenia about the right hip and a well-defined lytic area in the proximal femoral neck *(arrows)*.

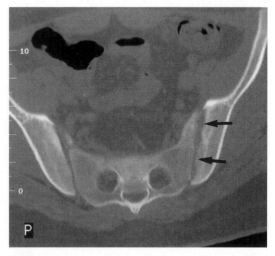

Figure 33–19. CT scan of patient with unilateral sacroiliitis as a result of presumed systemic arthritis *(arrows)*. The erosive changes of the left sacroiliac joint could not be seen on plain film.

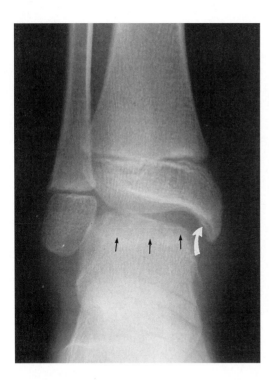

Figure 33–20. Hemophilic arthropathy of the ankle has resulted in erosion of the medial malleolus *(curved arrow)* and talar dome *(small arrows)*.

better formed in acquired dislocation (Fig. 33–22) than it is in developmental hip dysplasia, which facilitates the diagnosis.

Another condition, tarsal coalition, typically causes foot pain in the adolescent. It usually involves the talus and navicular bones (talonavicular coalition) or the talus and calcaneus (talocalcaneal coalition). The former is usually evaluated by plain foot radiographs and the latter by CT scan (Fig. 33–23).

Figure 33–21. Undiagnosed developmental dysplasia of both hips. The patient came to medical attention at 5 years of age. Both femoral heads are articulating with pseudoacetabulae *(arrows)*.

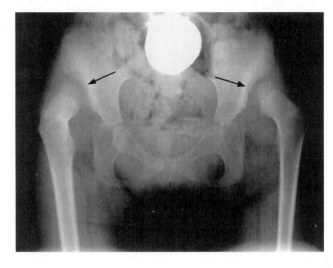

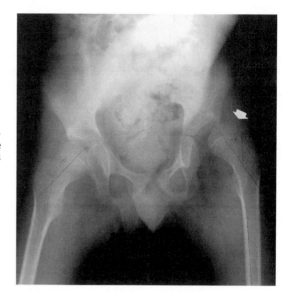

Figure 33–22. Acquired hip dislocation *(arrow)* in this neurologically impaired patient. The angles being measured are to assess coxa valga (the neck-shaft angle is too straight) as seen in patients who do not walk normally.

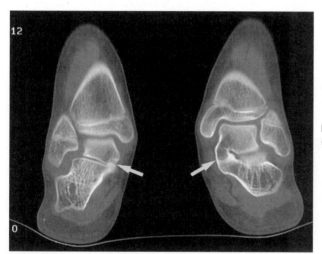

Figure 33–23. Bilateral talocalcaneal coalition *(arrows)* seen on CT scan.

Chapter 34

The Child with Back Pain

Back pain is an uncommon symptom in the pediatric patient. When it occurs, pathology is frequently present. The differential diagnosis of this entity includes trauma, tumors, infection/inflammation, normal variants resulting in abnormal stresses, and idiopathic conditions such as scoliosis and Scheuermann disease (idiopathic juvenile kyphosis).

RADIOGRAPHIC IMAGING

Imaging of children with back pain should always begin with spine radiographs. Frontal and lateral views are enough for screening. Oblique views can be done if pathology of the posterior elements is suspected. Assessing the normal spine involves evaluating for the normal lumbar lordosis. Its absence implies muscle spasm, as a general rule. Then the evaluation should include the vertebral bodies and their accompanying disc spaces. Finally, an evaluation of the neural arch or posterior elements should occur. The posterior elements are made up of pedicles, lamina, spinous processes, transverse processes, and superior and inferior articular processes. On the lateral view, the vertebral bodies should line up both anteriorly and posteriorly. Fusion anomalies should be sought. Klippel-Feil syndrome consists of any fusion anomaly of the cervical spine (Fig. 34–1). It is frequently associated with other anomalies such as vertebral anomalies further down and renal abnormalities. In the lumbar spine, the disc spaces should get wider as the spine is viewed inferiorly. The thoracic disc spaces should be uniform in thickness. In addition, the thoracic vertebral bodies should look more lucent as one proceeds inferiorly. If there is increased density, a lower lobe lung process is suspected (Fig. 34–2).

In the frontal view the pedicles should appear ovoid, and the distance between them (interpedic-

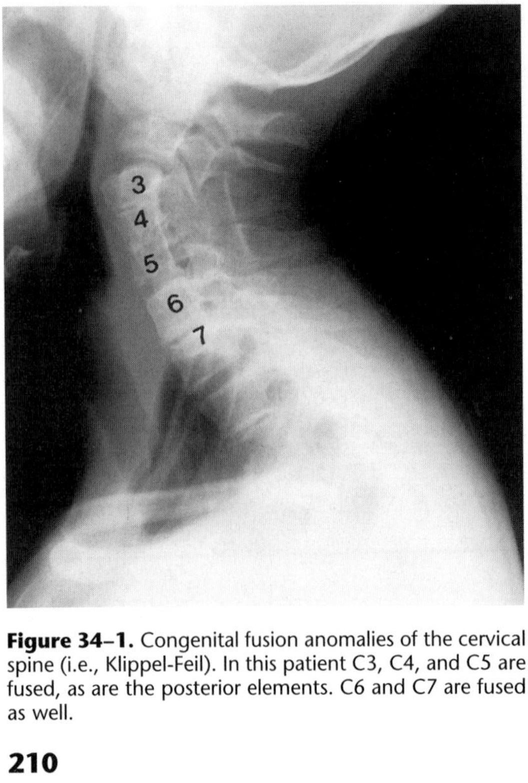

Figure 34–1. Congenital fusion anomalies of the cervical spine (i.e., Klippel-Feil). In this patient C3, C4, and C5 are fused, as are the posterior elements. C6 and C7 are fused as well.

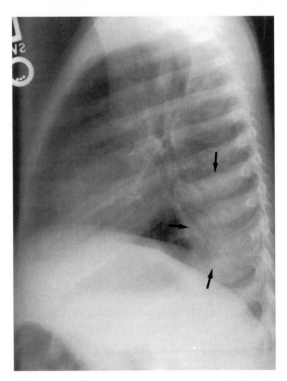

Figure 34–2. The density of the thoracic vertebral bodies increases as one goes inferiorly. Normally, there should be increased lucency. Therefore, a lower lobe lung process should be considered. In this case, right lower lobe pneumonia was present *(arrows)*.

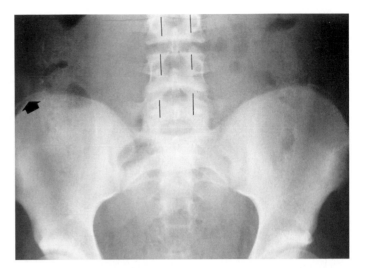

Figure 34–3. Lower normal lumbar spine. The vertical lines indicate the interpediculate distance. This distance gets slightly wider in the lumbar spine and narrows again in the sacral region. The arrow points out the normal mineralization of the iliac apophysis in this adolescent.

ulate distance) should be similar in the thoracic spine. It should be wide in the cervical spine and then widen slightly as the lumbar spine is scanned inferiorly (Fig. 34–3). The appearance of the posterior elements on the oblique view is similar to that of an animal and is frequently called the "Scotty dog." The neck of the dog, which is the pars interarticularis, should be carefully scrutinized for a fracture known as spondylolysis (Fig. 34–4). The presence of a spinous process at each level should be sought, although this structure is not ossified at birth. Its absence may indicate pathology, such as spina bifida. Usually spina bifida is associated with an abnormal appearance

of the pedicles in that they are thinner in the transverse plane, and the interpediculate distance is abnormally wide (Fig. 34–5).

In the neonate and young infant there may be a vertically oriented lucency seen on the lateral

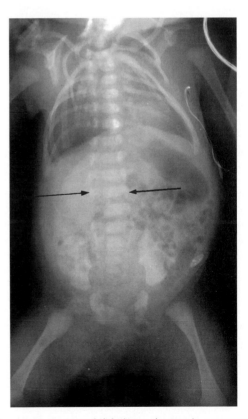

Figure 34–5. Spina bifida bony changes in a neonate. The interpediculate distance is abnormally wide, and the pedicles are narrow in the transverse dimension *(arrows)*.

Figure 34–4. Spondylolysis at L5 as seen by a fracture of the pars interarticularis (i.e., the "neck of the Scotty dog") *(open arrow)*. The neck of the vertebral Scotty dog above is intact *(curved arrow)*.

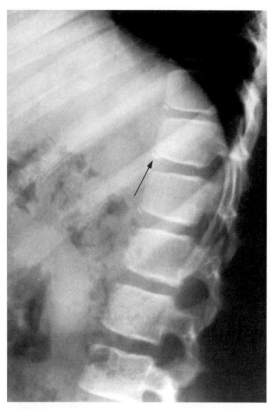

Figure 34–6. Normal ring apophyses *(arrow)* in the adolescent spine.

view in the vertebral body that is called a coronal cleft. This cleft is replaced by bone in infancy. In the adolescent spine, ossified ring apophyses (Fig. 34–6) can simulate corner fractures of the superior and inferior edges of the vertebral body. These fuse toward the end of puberty.

If no pathology is seen on plain radiographs or its presence is questionable, nuclear medicine bone scanning may be done to exclude occult pathology. CT scanning is the modality of choice for imaging the bony parts of the spine when an abnormality is suspected. MRI can be reserved for disc herniation or for spinal cord involvement when there is a fracture of the spinal column. It is also used for tumor evaluation because of its soft tissue detail and in some cases where inflammatory processes are present. MRI is sometimes used to evaluate marrow abnormality of the vertebral bodies.

TRAUMA

Acute traumatic injuries can result in various fractures of the vertebral column. Compression vertebral body fractures or separation of vertebral arches from their respective spinous processes can result when flexion stresses are placed on the spine. Extension stresses give fractures of the neural arches and widened disc spaces with "teardrop" fractures. In the acutely injured patient, plain film evaluation should start with cross-table lateral views of the entire spine. If a fracture is seen, the patient should have an unenhanced CT through the fracture and also through the vertebral bodies above and below this level to evaluate the stability of the lesion. A fracture involving both the vertebral body and the posterior elements is an unstable type of fracture. MRI can also be done to evaluate for possible cord involvement in the injury.

Cervical spine injuries in the patient under 8 years of age are usually confined to the C1–C2 region. The fractures most frequently occur through the synchondrosis of C2 (Fig. 34–7). Radiographic evaluation of the cervical spine should begin with the usual cross-table lateral view. An imaginary line connecting the front of the vertebral bodies, back of the bodies, and the spinous processes (spinolaminar line) should be visualized. With slight flexion there is slight movement of C2 on C3 ("pseudosubluxation") and inferiorly, but the spinolaminar line is still intact (Fig. 34–8).

The prevertebral soft tissues may be swollen with fractures. They should be no more than the anteroposterior width of C2 above the vocal cords, or 7 millimeters, and 14 millimeters below the vocal cords.

If the patient is taking medication such as exogenous steroids or has a malignancy such as leukemia that will result in diffuse osteopenia of the spine, compression vertebral body fractures can result from minor trauma (Fig. 34–9). These fractures are painful and may require bracing. Since the underlying bone is abnormal, these are pathologic fractures. Compression fractures involving normally mineralized bone result in increased density to the compressed vertebral body. Those that are pathologic will not result in increased sclerosis.

Spondylolysis

Chronic injury to the lumbar spine can result in fracture of the pars interarticularis (i.e., spondylolysis). This condition is most commonly seen in gymnasts who constantly flex and extend the lumbar spine. Controversy exists as to whether this condition results from a congenital predisposition or is acquired.

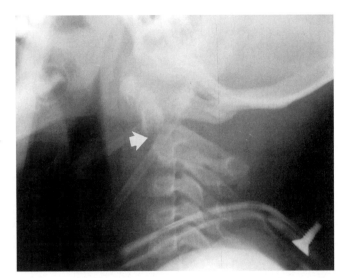

Figure 34–7. Fracture through the synchondrosis of C2 *(arrow).*

Initial evaluation with frontal and lateral views can make one suspect this condition, but oblique views of the spine will confirm it. The location of this abnormality is frequently at the L5-S1 level and is bilateral 75 to 80 percent of the time. On the oblique view, the fracture looks like the "neck of the Scotty dog" has been broken (Fig. 34–4). Sometimes the fracture might not be apparent, but the other side shows sclerosis because of abnormal stresses (Wilkinson syndrome). Nuclear medicine bone scanning with SPECT (which is like CT slices but in nuclear medicine) imaging

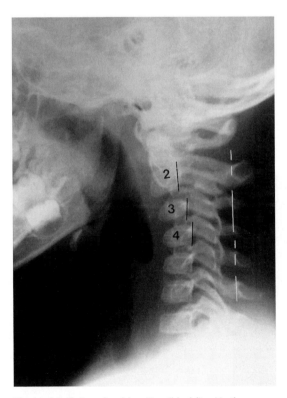

Figure 34–8. Pseudosubluxation *(black lines)* in the young child of C2 on C3 and C3 on C4. The spinolaminar line *(white lines)* is intact.

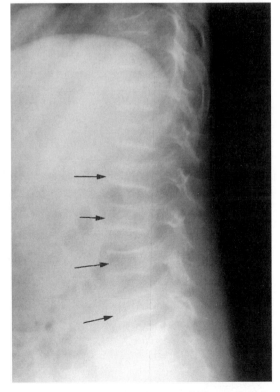

Figure 34–9. Patient with leukemia and diffuse pathologic compression fractures *(arrows).* The compressed bone is not sclerotic.

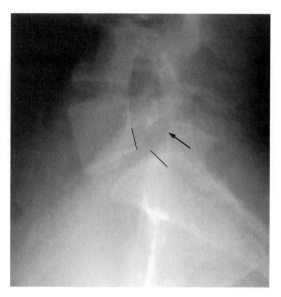

Figure 34–10. Spondylolisthesis of L5 and S1 due to bilateral spondylolysis *(arrow)*. L5 is anterior to S1 as shown by the black lines.

can sometimes be used to diagnose this condition. When the condition is bilateral, the involved vertebral body can slip anteriorly upon the one beneath it, a condition called spondylolisthesis (Fig. 34–10).

TUMORS

Tumors of the bony elements of the vertebral column as well as tumors involving the spinal cord itself can cause back pain. Those in the bone could be benign or malignant and could cause a painful scoliosis. Idiopathic scoliosis is usually not painful.

Benign Bony Tumors

Osteoid Osteoma. The most common location of an osteoid osteoma arising in the spine is from the posterior elements, usually a pedicle. The plain film findings in this condition are that of a sclerotic lesion with a lucent center. The lucent center is the actual vascular tumor, which is surrounded by reactive sclerosis. The lesion shows intense radiotracer uptake on nuclear medicine bone scan. If further imaging is required preoperatively, CT scan with thin slices is helpful for further localization.

Osteoblastoma. Osteoblastoma is a giant osteoid osteoma larger than 2 centimeters that also frequently arises from the posterior elements of the spine. The lesion has a tendency to grow and cause cortical expansion with reactive sclerosis around it. The tumor nidus is also large. Like the osteoid osteoma, the nuclear medicine bone scan shows intense uptake in the lesion.

Aneurysmal Bone Cyst. An aneurysmal bone cyst is another benign tumor of the posterior elements that causes an expansile lesion with a thin rim of cortical bone around it unless there has been a pathologic fracture through it. Either CT or MRI should be used to image this lesion. Bone scan will only show a "cold" area surrounded by minimally increased activity. CT will show the bony expansion well and may show the fluid-fluid level that is characteristic of the inside of this lesion (Fig. 34–11). MRI shows the fluid-fluid levels to a greater degree, but rarely are both imaging modalities necessary.

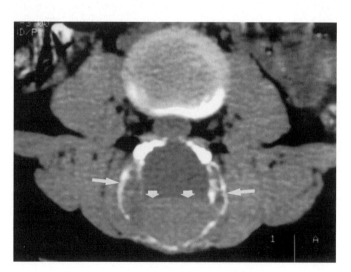

Figure 34–11. CT scan of an aneurysmal bone cyst of the spinous process *(long arrows)* with the characteristic fluid-fluid level *(broad arrows)*.

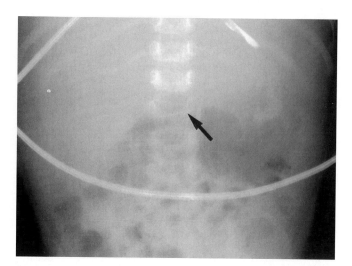

Figure 34–12. Histiocytosis involvement of L2 vertebral body with asymmetric compression of the body *(arrow)* and increased lucency compared with the other vertebral bodies.

Malignant Bone Tumors

Langerhans Cell Histiocytosis. Langerhans cell histiocytosis is a process involving the medullary canal of bone with histiocyte proliferation that goes to any bone but can involve the vertebral column, most commonly the vertebral body (Fig. 34–12). The classic appearance of this process in the vertebral body is diffuse osteopenia with vertebral body compression fractures sometimes so involved that the body is completely collapsed (i.e., vertebral plana).

In other bones the lesions are lytic with no sclerosis around them. When the calvarium is involved, the edge of the lesion has a beveled edge due to the location of the lesion within the diploic space and erosion of the inner and outer table to a different degree (Fig. 34–13). Unlike a lot of bony processes, nuclear medicine bone scan is not useful in this diagnosis since these lesions are lytic and the bone scan usually cannot resolve them. Plain films are the way to diagnose and follow these lesions.

Ewing Sarcoma. Other primary malignant bone tumors besides histiocytosis are unusual. However, Ewing sarcoma is the most frequently encountered. The sacrum is more commonly involved than are other parts of the spine. Plain film diagnosis can be difficult when the lesion is in the sacrum since this area is difficult to see radiographically because of overlying stool and gas in the bowel. MRI is best at evaluating the soft tissue involvement, especially the spinal canal invasion. CT can show the bony destruction, if necessary, but this modality is chiefly used to diagnose lung metastases.

Metastases. Malignant tumors involving the spine are usually metastatic from small, round, blue cell tumors (as seen histologically) such as leukemia, neuroblastoma, Ewing sarcoma, and medulloblastoma. With the exception of medulloblastoma, these metastases are usually lytic processes. Leukemia can cause diffuse osteopenia as well, which can result in compression vertebral body fractures (Fig. 34–9).

Spinal Cord Tumors. The most frequently encountered spinal cord tumor is an astrocytoma, which is most often found in the cervical spine

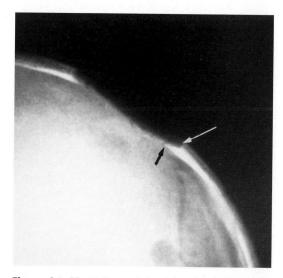

Figure 34–13. Histiocytosis involving the skull. A close-up view showing the lesion in the diploic space that is eroding the inner *(black arrow)* and outer *(white arrow)* table to different degrees.

region. Plain films may show an abnormally widened interpediculate distance. However, this is a difficult diagnosis to make in this region because the cervical spine normally has widening of the interpediculate distance. MRI is the imaging modality of choice for this diagnosis because of its exquisite resolution of the spinal cord.

INFECTION AND INFLAMMATION

Discitis

Discitis is discussed in Chapter 8. It can occur in the adolescent and cause changes similar to those seen in the young child (Fig. 34–14).

Tuberculosis

Tuberculosis is becoming more common. Although rarely seen in the pediatric patient, tuberculosis can infect the spine (Pott disease) by being carried as a blood-borne pathogen with invasion of the vertebrae and subsequent infection of the disc via communicating vessels through the vertebral endplate. Plain films can show destruction of both the disc space and the surrounding vertebral bodies (Fig. 34–15). In addition, the presence of a paraspinous mass due to soft-tissue abscess

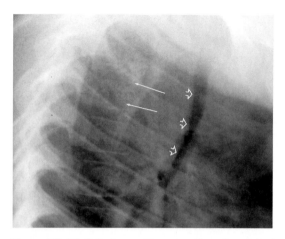

Figure 34–15. Pott disease. The upper thoracic vertebral bodies are difficult to see because of destruction by TB *(long arrows)*. There is a mediastinal mass present, as well, with anterior bowing of the trachea *(open arrows)*.

formation can be detected. CT is helpful in visualizing the bony involvement, and MRI can visualize the bone marrow involvement as well as the soft tissue component.

IDIOPATHIC CONDITIONS

Transitional Vertebral Bodies

Transitional vertebral bodies are congenital normal variants that are usually seen at the L5-S1 level. On plain films of this region, the lowest lumbar vertebra may have the appearance of being part of the sacrum without a clear-cut disc space (sacralization) or the first sacral segment may look like a lumbar vertebral body (lumbarization). This congenital variant can place abnormal stresses on the involved vertebral bodies and result in low back pain.

Scheuermann Disease

Scheuermann disease is also known as juvenile thoracic kyphosis. This condition is more common in males and occurs at the onset of puberty. On plain lateral spine radiographs, there is vertebral endplate irregularity caused by herniation of the nucleus pulposus into the vertebral body. This is known as Schmorl nodes. In addition, there is anterior wedging of the vertebral bodies and narrowing of the intervertebral disc spaces (Fig. 34–16). The condition usually affects three or more contiguous vertebral bodies and is most commonly present in the midthoracic and upper lumbar spine. Nuclear medicine bone scanning is

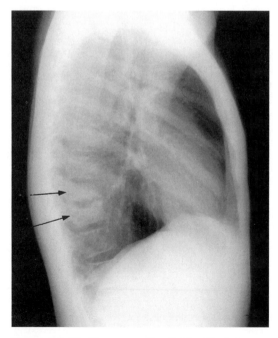

Figure 34–14. Teenager with discitis. *Staphylococcus aureus* was cultured from the inflammatory mass around the involved vertebral bodies *(arrows)*.

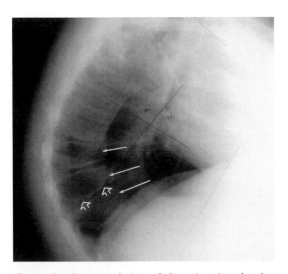

Figure 34–16. Lateral view of thoracic spine showing excessive kyphosis (>40 degrees) with anterior wedging of at least three contiguous vertebral bodies *(long arrows)*. The endplates of these vertebral bodies are irregular *(open arrows)*.

normal in this condition. Other imaging modalities are not necessary. Treatment is with an orthopedic brace and, occasionally, fusion rods.

Scoliosis

Scoliosis is sometimes associated with back pain because of abnormal stress placed on certain parts of the spine as a result of the curve. There are several types of scoliosis.

Congenital scoliosis results from a vertebral anomaly (Fig. 34–17) such as a hemivertebra or block vertebra. A block vertebra is due to congenital fusion of two or more vertebral bodies. An abnormal bony bridge connecting a portion of two or more vertebral bodies, known as a vertebral bar formation, is a type of partial block vertebra formation.

Neurologically abnormal children have a C-shaped curve due to the abnormal and umbalanced muscle pull seen in these patients (Fig. 34–18). The idiopathic type is frequently S-shaped. This idiopathic type is divided into three different types: infantile, juvenile, and adolescent.

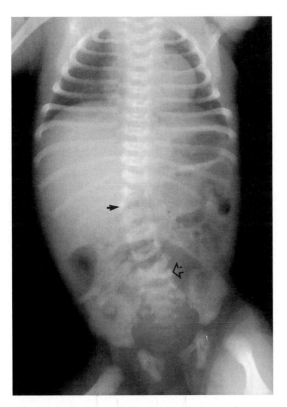

Figure 34–17. Congenital scoliosis with vertebral anomalies at T12 level and L5 level. The upper anomaly consists of an extra pedicle *(closed arrow)*, and the lower is a hemivertebra *(open arrow)*.

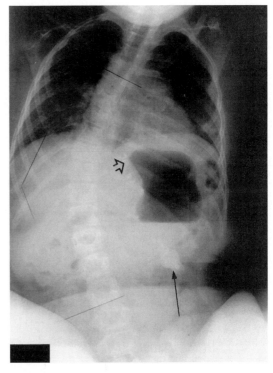

Figure 34–18. C-shaped neuromuscular curve in this patient with cerebral palsy. Note the gastrostomy tube *(long arrow)* and clips from an antireflux procedure *(open arrow)*.

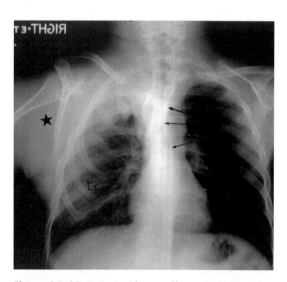

Figure 34–19. Patient with neurofibromatosis. There is a short, angled curve *(long arrows)*. Also present are abnormally thinned, ribbony, ribs anteriorly *(open arrow)* and a large neurofibrosarcoma involving the right shoulder *(star)*.

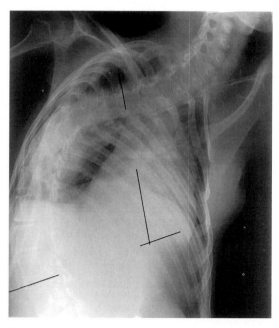

Figure 34–20. Measuring the C-shaped curve by the Cobb method as demonstrated by the black lines.

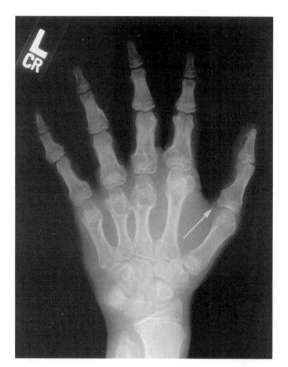

Figure 34–21. Left hand in a male patient with multiple exostoses that has a bone age of at least 13 years because the adductor sesamoid *(arrow)* is present.

Patients with underlying syndromes can have scoliosis as a manifestation of their condition. Marfan syndrome and neurofibromatosis are two such entities. The scoliosis seen with neurofibromatosis is typically short and acutely angled (Fig. 34–19). That seen in Marfan syndrome can be identical to the idiopathic variety, but it occurs at an earlier age and typically is more severe. Scoliosis, regardless of the type, is best evaluated on plain radiographs. The frontal view of the entire spine with the patient either sitting or standing is the preferred film. The curve is measured by the Cobb method (Fig. 34–20). This method involves finding the vertebral body where the curve begins and ends, drawing horizontal lines parallel to these vertebral bodies, and then dropping perpendicular lines from these horizontal ones and forming an angle. More than 10 degrees is considered scoliosis.

In patients being assessed for surgical repair of their curve, an estimation of skeletal maturation is done. It is desirable to correct the curve in a patient that is as skeletally mature as possible due to the fusion of the spine that occurs with the correction, which does not allow for more growth.

Two methods of skeletal maturation can be done. The first involves comparing the frontal view of the left hand with the standards of Greulich and Pyle. They have compiled an atlas of left hands showing development of the neonatal hand compared to that seen at skeletal maturity. To assess skeletal maturity, the patient's left hand radiograph is compared with the atlas pictures. Matching the terminal phalangeal epiphyses first is the most accurate. Once these epiphyseal centers have been matched, comparison with the more proximal centers should be done. If the patient's skeletal maturation falls within two standard deviations, it is considered within the normal range. An anatomic landmark, the adductor sesamoid of the thumb, appears characteristically at age 11 in females and at age 13 in males (Fig. 34–21).

The second method is called the Risser method. This method involves an assessment of ossification of the iliac apophysis. It is the last to fuse in the skeleton. When the apophysis appears, it ossifies in a lateral to medial direction and is graded from zero to five (Fig. 34–3), where five is compete fusion and zero indicates it has not appeared.

Sometimes other imaging modalities, usually MRI, are needed if the curve is unusual in any way or if an underlying bony or soft-tissue process is suspected to be causing the curve. For example, a patient that has spina bifida and develops scoliosis frequently has either an underlying cord abnormality (common in this disorder) or has tethering of the cord in the repair of the original myelomeningocele. MRI is recommended in these patients before scoliosis surgery is performed.

Chapter 35

The Older Infant and Child with Bowed Lower Extremities

In the evaluation of this problem, plain radiographs of the lower extremities with the patient standing are usually sufficient for diagnosis. However, if these films suggest an underlying skeletal dysplasia, an entire skeletal survey should be performed not only to confirm the diagnosis but also to assess the degree of skeletal involvement. Anytime an underlying syndrome is suspected, a good text on syndromes is a must.

In the differential diagnosis of bowed lower extremities, there are many possibilities: Blount disease (idiopathic tibia vara), physiologic bowing, old traumatic deformity, osteogenesis imperfecta, fibrous dysplasia, rickets, and multiple enchondromatosis, among others. The first three diagnoses only need the lower extremities radiographed to diagnose the condition, but the other diagnoses frequently need a skeletal survey for confirmation.

BLOUNT DISEASE

Blount disease is seen in two age ranges: the toddler who is just beginning to ambulate and the adolescent. These children are usually overweight and very bowlegged (genu varus) clinically. The entity is an avascular necrosis of the medial tibial metaphysis. Plain radiographs show irregularity of the proximal medial tibial metaphysis. There is sclerosis of this area and of the area distal to this in the metadiaphyseal region (Fig. 35–1). As a result of this deformity the proximal tibial epiphysis is dysplastic, and the tibial articular surface displays a medial downward sloping angle. The medial femoral condyle also is affected and demonstrates dysplasia as a result. Treatment of severe disease is surgical with creation of a valgus-producing osteotomy of the proximal tibia. Blount disease must be distinguished from physiologic bowing.

PHYSIOLOGIC BOWING OF THE LOWER EXTREMITIES

Physiologic bowing has no dysplasia of the bones. Specifically, the proximal tibial metaphysis is not irregular and sclerotic. There is no medial downward sloping of the articular surface of the tibia. With time, the bowlegged feature usually gets better.

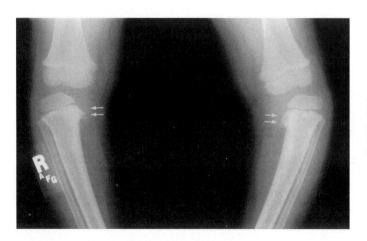

Figure 35–1. Blount disease seen in this toddler. The medial tibial metaphysis (arrows) is the site of the abnormality that results in the genu varus deformity bilaterally.

POSTTRAUMATIC DEFORMITY

Old traumatic deformity can result in bowing of the lower extremities. If the proximal tibial growth plate is injured and prematurely fuses medially, then the tibia appears bowed. More often a fracture of the proximal tibia, not involving the physis, can result in a valgus deformity.

OSTEOGENESIS IMPERFECTA

Osteogenesis imperfecta (OI) is usually already diagnosed by the time the patient is a young child. In this entity the bones are unusually fragile and result in microfractures and visible fractures with bowing occurring over time. Overall mineralization is usually decreased so that the bones are more lucent than normal (Fig. 35–2). If the diagnosis has not been made before, a skeletal survey should complete the evaluation. Wormian bones (intrasutural bones), seen best in the lambdoidal suture of the skull, should be sought. Greater than 10 wormian bones supports the diagnosis of OI, together with the finding of diffuse osteopenia, bony deformity, and the presence or absence of fractures.

FIBROUS DYSPLASIA

Fibrous dysplasia can affect a single bone or multiple bones as diagnosed on a skeletal survey. The lesions are well defined and present in the medullary cavity of the affected bones. The texture of the lesion has been described as having a "ground-glass" appearance. Patients usually present with pathologic fractures. Because these lesions are vascular, there can be overgrowth as well as bowing deformity of the affected extremity. The lower extremity is frequently affected and there is resultant leg-length discrepancy. Bone scanning, although usually only necessary to diagnose the solitary lesions, shows increased activity uniformly (Fig. 35–3). When fibrous dysplasia involves multiple sites in a unilateral fashion and is associated with precocious puberty in females, the syndrome is called McCune-Albright syndrome.

RICKETS

Rickets is osteomalacia of growing bone. Osteomalacia occurs when there is an excessive amount of uncalcified osteoid and insufficient mineralization of osteoid. This process causes bones to be softer than normal, resulting in bowing if not treated (Fig. 35–4). Radiographically,

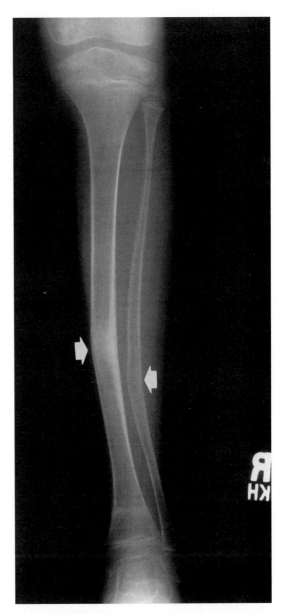

Figure 35–2. Patient with osteogenesis imperfecta with diffuse osteopenia and bowing deformity from previous fractures *(arrows)*.

rickets resulting from any etiology looks the same. The earliest radiographic sign of rickets is loss of the normal white line at the edge of the metaphysis, followed by apparent widening of the physis, and then there is cupping and fraying of the metaphysis (Fig. 35–5). The areas to manifest rickets or any other metabolic bone disease are the fastest growing areas, namely, the knees, ankles, hands, and wrists. Only frontal views of these areas are

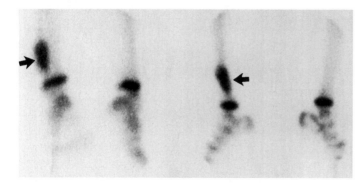

Figure 35–3. Isolated lesion of fibrous dysplasia in the distal fibula *(arrows)*. Because of its intensely vascular nature, the bone scan is quite ''hot'' The lesion caused a varus bowing of the distal fibula.

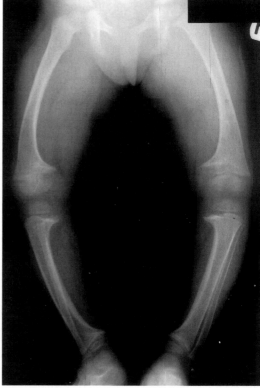

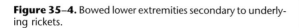

Figure 35–4. Bowed lower extremities secondary to underlying rickets.

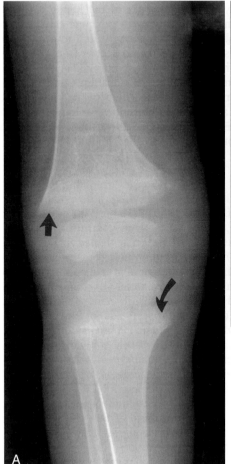

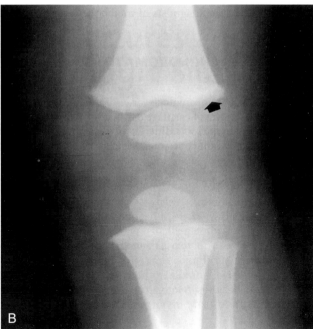

Figure 35–5. A, Rickets in the knee with widening of the physis, metaphyseal flaring *(curved arrow)* and fraying *(straight arrow).* **B,** Normal knee with dense, white line of the metaphysis *(arrow).*

Figure 35–6. Multiple enchondromatosis seen throughout the pelvis and proximal femurs. The lesions in the proximal left femur have caused a varus bowing of the femoral neck *(arrows).*

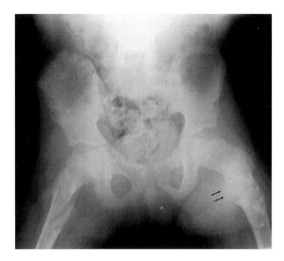

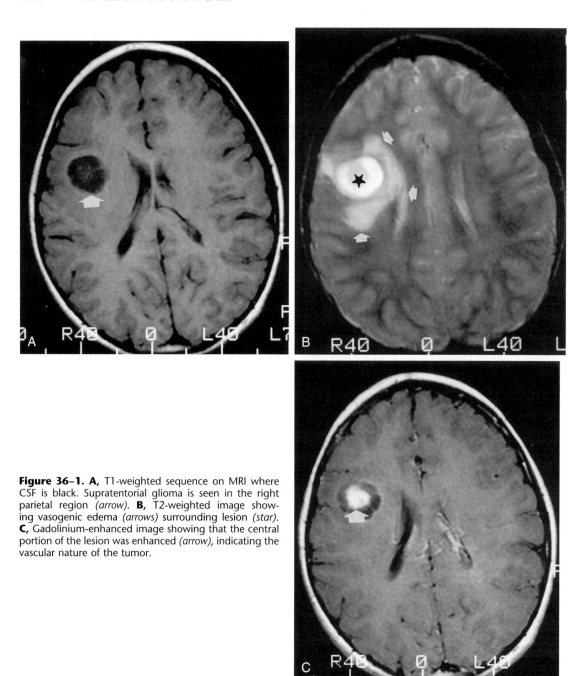

Figure 36–1. A, T1-weighted sequence on MRI where CSF is black. Supratentorial glioma is seen in the right parietal region *(arrow)*. **B,** T2-weighted image showing vasogenic edema *(arrows)* surrounding lesion *(star)*. **C,** Gadolinium-enhanced image showing that the central portion of the lesion was enhanced *(arrow)*, indicating the vascular nature of the tumor.

In general, accidental fractures in children less than 2 years of age are frequently linear in appearance and parietal in location. Depressed skull fractures are more common as the patient becomes older. Leptomeningeal cysts are a complication of skull fractures that occur in patients less than 3 years of age. The cysts are caused when the skull fracture tears through the dura with herniation of arachnoid tissue through the dural defect. The constant pulsation of brain tissue against the skull erodes the calvarium over time. The underlying brain usually demonstrates encephalomalacia. If plain films are obtained, the previous fracture margins are widely separated and show scalloping

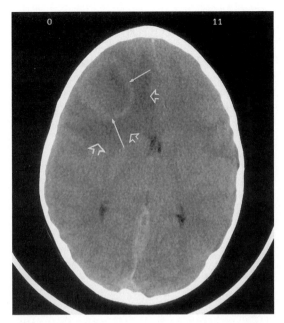

Figure 36–2. Brain abscess *(long arrows)* with surrounding edema *(open arrows)* and resulting mass effect with shift of the midline from right to left. The abscess was a result of frontal sinusitis.

at their edges (Fig. 36–3). CT or MRI can demonstrate the underlying area of encephalomalacia.

An incidental finding that can be seen on the initial trauma cross-table lateral cervical spine is an air-fluid level in the sphenoid sinus. This finding is indicative of a basilar skull fracture in the setting of trauma (Fig. 36–4).

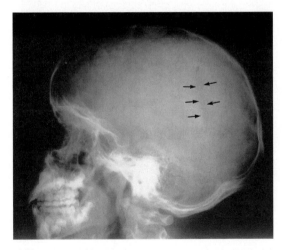

Figure 36–3. Leptomeningeal cyst. A "growing" fracture *(arrows)* in a pediatric patient due to an associated tear in the underlying dura with subsequent pulsation of the underlying brain against the skull fracture.

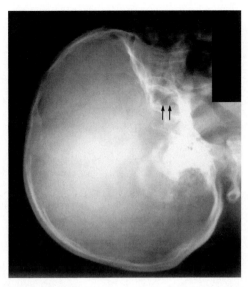

Figure 36–4. Air-fluid level in sphenoid sinus *(arrows)* taken on cross-table lateral view indicative of a basilar skull fracture.

Hematomas

Hematomas can be subdural, epidural, intracerebral, and subarachnoid. Most subdural hematomas are located in a supratentorial location. If the patient is less than 1 year of age, shaken infant syndrome is the most likely diagnosis. CT evaluation of a subdural hematoma shows a crescentic fluid collection that is of high attenuation for several days after the injury (Fig. 30–8). Then the collection becomes isodense with the brain and, subsequently, becomes hypointense and looks similar to CSF. MRI is more sensitive than CT for viewing the subdural collections. In addition, MRI is useful for determining the age of the collections when there is more than one and when the collection has the same attenuation as CSF on CT scan.

Epidural hematomas are usually parietal or temporal in location and 40 percent are associated with fractures. On CT the collection is convex medially (Fig. 36–5) with the appearance of attenuation values being the same as with other blood collections.

Intracerebral blood collections are associated with fractures in two thirds and most often have frontal and parietal locations. Another cause for intracerebral blood is a ruptured aneurysm, which is rare in the pediatric patient.

Subarachnoid hemorrhage is best evaluated on CT because it can be missed with MRI. To diagnose subarachnoid hemorrhage, increased attenuation in the cisterns and along the sylvian fissures

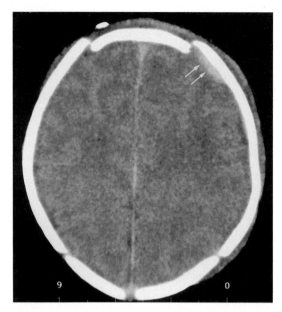

Figure 36–5. Extraaxial (outside brain substance) acute blood in this young infant *(arrows)*. It has a convex medial border indicating that it is an epidural hematoma.

is seen. When the blood collects along the falx, there is irregularity of that structure. This diagnosis can be simulated in the young brain. Normally the immature brain is of low attenuation because of the high water content. This appearance causes normal vascular structures to appear at higher attenuation values and can simulate extravascular blood.

Cerebral Edema

Cerebral edema is also seen in the setting of trauma. CT is the best modality for evaluating this entity in the acute traumatic setting. When cerebral edema is present, there is poor delineation of the white matter and cortex with obliteration of the cisterns (Fig. 36–6). Cerebral edema takes approximately 8 to 12 hours to show up on a CT scan. When it is present, it can persist for 2 to 3 days. When it is severe, diffusely low attenuation to the supratentorial structures as compared to the posterior fossa is frequently seen. This finding is called the "white cerebellum" sign, which is usually associated with a poor outcome (Fig. 36–7). In patients who have so much cerebral edema, there will be total obstruction of intracranial blood flow resulting in brain death. This

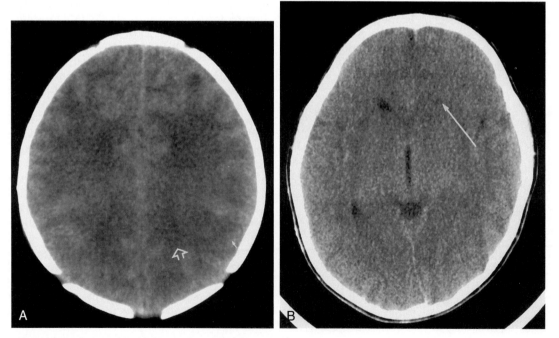

Figure 36–6. A, Normal newborn with delineation of both gray *(small arrow)* and white *(open arrow)* matter. **B,** Older child with cerebral edema in which all brain substance is of one attenuation value. The ventricles are becoming obliterated *(arrow).*

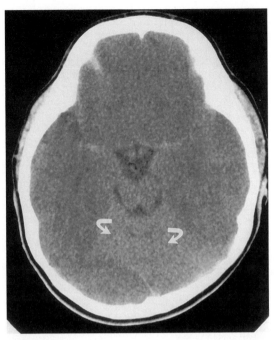

Figure 36–7. "White cerebellum" sign, in which the infratentorial structures *(curved arrows)* are of higher attenuation value than are the supratentorial structures, indicating cerebral edema and frequently a poor outcome.

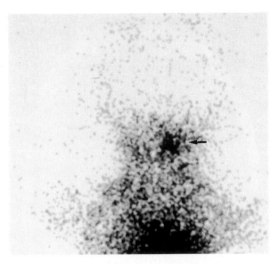

Figure 36–8. Brain death with radiopharmaceutical seen only in the external carotid circulation: "hot nose" phenomenon *(arrow)*.

phenomenon is best imaged with a nuclear medicine brain flow study. The study involves injection of a radiopharmaceutical and the imaging of the tracer over the head and neck. The blood is diverted into the external carotid circulation ("hot nose") because of the elevated intracranial pressure (Fig. 36–8).

Foreign Bodies

Foreign bodies in the brain can be assessed by both plain film and CT. Remember that metallic foreign bodies in the brain or orbit are contraindications to MRI. The brain does not scar in or around the foreign bodies, and orbital metallic foreign bodies can move in the magnetic field, resulting in blindness.

CNS VASCULAR ABNORMALITIES

Cerebrovascular Accidents

Cerebrovascular accidents (CVA) are unusual in the pediatric population, but, when present, they are frequently associated with underlying problems such as sickle cell disease, vasculitis, severe hypotension, and cocaine abuse. In the

initial stages of a CVA the CT scan may be normal or may show edematous changes in the arterial distribution of the occluded artery (Fig. 36–9). Later, there will be atrophic changes with ipsilateral dilatation of the lateral ventricle if the area of infarction is large enough. MRI is more sensitive for diagnosing the early changes of focal edema than is CT. MR angiography can be done to see the vascular lesion and may negate the need for cerebral angiography.

Arteriovenous Malformations

Aneurysms of the brain are rare in children, so they will not be discussed. Arteriovenous malformations (AVMs) are more common and usually present with bleeding before the patient is 20 years of age. Eighty percent of all AVMs are supratentorial. Imaging of them is most efficiently performed with MRI or with contrast-enhanced CT scanning. The MRI shows the tortuous veins to be of low signal intensity because of the flowing blood unless there is clotting in the AVM. MRI is usually the preferred imaging modality over enhanced CT scanning because of the radiation involved and the potential risks encountered in the use of intravenous contrast. The vein of Galen malformation is an important AVM that presents in the neonatal period 90 percent of the time and causes the patient to be in high-output congestive heart failure. Occasionally this malformation will be detected later because of hydrocephalus and seizures, which can occur. Sometimes these AVMs

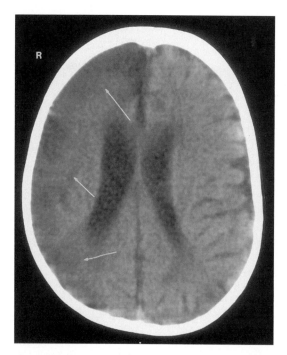

Figure 36–9. Cerebral infarction on the right in the middle cerebral artery distribution *(arrows)*. The sulcation is effaced on this side indicating edema. This suggests that the infarct is not old.

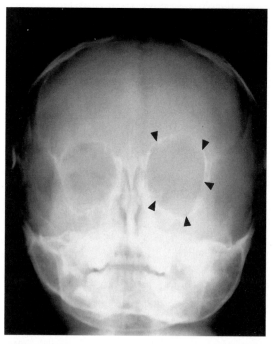

Figure 36–10. Patient with neurofibromatosis with enlargement of the left orbit and abnormal lucency in the orbit due to hypoplasia of the sphenoid *(arrowheads)*.

are found incidentally when they have spontaneously thrombosed and calcified. They are located in the posterior incisura region and sometimes elevate the third ventricle.

NEUROCUTANEOUS SYNDROMES

Neurocutaneous syndromes, as the name implies, are syndromes that have skin lesions coexistent with neurological abnormalities. The most common syndromes are neurofibromatosis and tuberous sclerosis. Less common are those that involve vascular abnormalities and include Sturge-Weber syndrome, Von-Hippel-Lindau disease, ataxia-telangiectasia, among others.

Neurofibromatosis

Neurofibromatosis consists of two types. It is type 1, however, that is most frequently seen in children. It involves the nervous system as well as the skeletal system and skin. The most common manifestation of neurofibromatosis in the skeleton is scoliosis, which is often an acute and short curve, as was mentioned in Chapter 34. Other

manifestations are ribbonlike ribs, posterior scalloping of the vertebral bodies, focal overgrowth of a digit, tibial pseudarthrosis, hypoplasia of the lesser wing of the sphenoid in the skull (Fig. 36–10), and asymmetry of the optic foramen due to optic nerve tumors, among others. Imaging of these skeletal abnormalities is best done with a skeletal survey.

The brain parenchymal abnormalities are optic nerve gliomas, which are seen most often in the first decade. MRI is the most sensitive imaging modality to detect these tumors, as well as metastases in the brain. Other tumors and masses seen are the soft-tissue neurofibromas, lateral meningoceles, schwannomas, and pheochromocytomas. For tumors and masses involving the spinal cord, MRI is the most often used imaging modality.

Tuberous Sclerosis

Tuberous sclerosis is another neuroectodermal disorder that is characterized by skin lesions, such as adenoma sebaceum, seizures, and mental retardation. In the brain the lesions seen are hamartomas, giant cell astrocytomas, and heterotopic is-

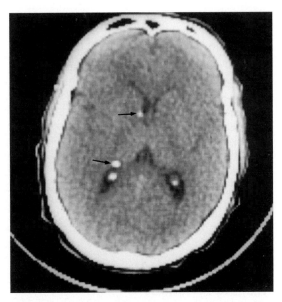

Figure 36–11. Old-fashioned unenhanced CT scan of patient with tuberous sclerosis showing periventricular calcifications *(arrows)*. The other calcific densities in the ventricles are calcified choroid plexuses.

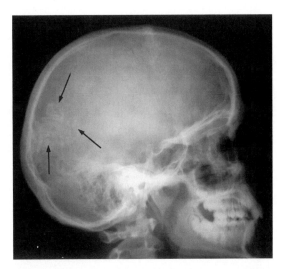

Figure 36–12. The "tram track" calcification *(arrows)* seen with Sturge-Weber syndrome.

lands of gray matter in the white matter. The hamartomas are located in the subependymal area of the cortex and are frequently calcified. Giant cell astrocytomas are located near the foramen of Monro. Heterotopic islands of gray matter can be located anywhere in the white matter. Imaging is best with MRI, although the calcification is best seen on unenhanced CT. The CT scan has usually been done prior to a lumbar puncture and shows periventricular calcification (Fig. 36–11). The lesions on MRI are frequently hyperintense on T2-weighted images.

Other organs that may be involved in tuberous sclerosis include the kidneys, heart, lung, and skeleton. In the kidneys, renal cysts and angiomyolipomas are most common and can be imaged on ultrasound first, then followed by abdominal CT if necessary. On ultrasound the angiomyolipomas are echogenic because of the fat they contain. The heart shows multiple rhabdomyomas resulting clinically in arrhythmias. These lesions are first seen on cardiac echo and the diagnosis is confirmed, if necessary, by biopsy. The lungs show an interstitial pattern particularly in the lower lungs and can be associated with a spontaneous pneumothorax and chylous pleural effusion. Plain chest radiograph is the best modality for imaging these findings. The skeletal involvement shows sclerotic patches most frequently involving the calvarium. There also can be periosteal thickening of the long bones and bone cysts in the distal phalanges. All these bony findings are best seen on skeletal survey.

Sturge-Weber Syndrome

Sturge-Weber syndrome is also called encephalotrigeminal angiomatosis and is associated with seizures, mental retardation, congenital unilateral facial port wine stain, and angiomas of the leptomeninges. The port wine stain is present in the distribution of the first and second divisions of the fifth cranial nerve. Angiomas of the leptomeninges are seen most commonly in the parietal region and are associated with hemiatrophy of the brain beneath the angiomas and calcifications of the brain in a gyriform pattern underlying the vascular lesion. Plain skull radiographs are classic in patients over 2 years of age with the calcification seen in a "tram track" pattern (Fig. 36–12). The calcifications are also seen on CT. MRI can be done, but it usually is not necessary because the diagnosis is readily made based on the physical examination.

Von Hippel-Lindau Disease

Von Hippel-Lindau disease involves hemangioblastomas of all organs but most commonly the CNS. On CT these lesions are large and cystic appearing with a mural nodule that enhances with intravenous contrast material. On MRI the cystic component is hyperintense on T2-weighted images, as is the mural nodule. CNS involvement is the most frequent cause of morbidity and mortality in this syndrome. Early on, the kidneys can be involved with cortical cysts, which are best seen on ultrasound. There is a predisposition to renal cell carcinoma in the older patient. The adrenal gland may demonstrate a pheochromocytoma.

Ataxia Telangiectasia

Ataxia telangiectasia is a disorder characterized by cerebellar ataxia, pulmonary infections, immunodeficiencies, mucocutaneous telangiectasias, and a propensity to develop malignancies such as lymphoma. The patient has a progressive neurologic deterioration and also has recurrent infections. CT of the brain shows cerebellar atrophy as manifested by decreased cerebellar size and increased prominence to the cerebellar sulci.

MASS LESIONS OTHER THAN NEOPLASMS

Mass lesions, as well as neoplasms, can frequently present with seizures. Mass lesions can be cysts, either arachnoid cysts or porencephalic cysts. Cysts due to echinococcus are rarely seen. Porencephalic cysts are areas of encephalomalacia that communicate with the ventricle most of the time, but they can enlarge if they do not communicate. Etiology of these porencephalic areas can be congenital or acquired, with the latter usually a result of intracranial bleeding, infarction, or infection. Unenhanced CT shows areas of decreased attenuation similar to that of CSF but located in the brain parenchyma. Arachnoid cysts are extraaxial (outside the brain substance) and have a mass effect on surrounding structures. As a result, treatment usually involves shunting the cyst. Etiology of these cysts is congenital as a result of the division of the arachnoid membrane with expansion of CSF due to the secretory activity of arachnoid cells. These arachnoid cysts are seen 50 percent of the time in the sylvian fissure.

Imaging of the cysts can easily be accomplished by head ultrasound if there is still a patent anterior fontanel that will allow a transducer head to be used for imaging. If there is none, both unenhanced CT and unenhanced MRI can be used to evaluate the cyst and surrounding structures. MRI is particularly good because multiple imaging planes can be obtained.

NEOPLASMS

Fifty to sixty percent of all neoplasms are gliomas. The gliomas consist of astrocytomas, peripheral neuroectodermal tumors (PNET), and ependymomas. Location of the lesions is divided between supratentorial and infratentorial regions. The most common supratentorial lesion is the cerebral astrocytoma followed by the optic nerve glioma. The most common infratentorial lesion is the cerebellar astrocytoma, which is followed by PNET/medulloblastoma, and then by brain stem glioma. All the various mass lesions are best seen on MRI, both unenhanced and enhanced. Frequently, an unenhanced CT scan will be the first imaging modality because it is done as a screening procedure.

Imaging of Tumors

The radiographic appearance of the cerebellar astrocytoma classically is a cystic mass with a mural nodule that has little surrounding edema and is located in the cerebellar hemisphere. On MRI the cystic component is hyperintense on T2-weighted images. The mural nodule is hyperintense on the same imaging sequence with inhomogeneous enhancement of the tumor nodule. The cystic component enhances little, if any.

Peripheral neuroectodermal tumors are undifferentiated tumors that resemble the medulloblastoma histologically and arise from almost anywhere but cannot otherwise be classified into recognizable histologic categories. Only the supratentorial undifferentiated tumor will be discussed here. Imaging of these lesions often reveals a large hemispheric mass with calcification or a cystic component. The appearance on both CT and MRI is variable with contrast enhancement commonly seen with either modality.

Medulloblastoma (PNET arising in the cerebellum) arises in the midline from the cerebellar vermis and grows into the fourth ventricle. The tumor infiltrates the cerebellar hemispheres and spreads through CSF spaces to the surfaces of neural structures. This tumor is the most common childhood tumor producing intracranial and intraspinal seeding. Imaging is most often performed with MRI, which shows intense contrast enhancement but is variable in appearance with the various imaging sequences. There is usually high intensity edema surrounding the lesion. CT, which is sometimes performed first, frequently shows a hyperdense lesion because of its high cellular content (Fig. 36–

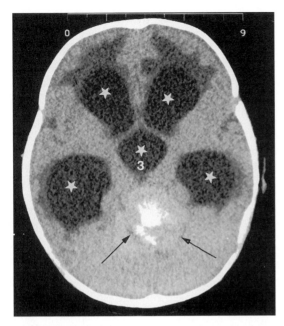

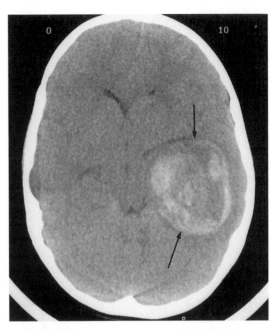

Figure 36–13. CT scan of medulloblastoma *(arrows),* which is obliterating the fourth ventricle as well as the aqueduct, resulting in marked ventricular dilation of the third and lateral ventricles *(stars).*

Figure 36–14. CT scan of supratentorial left temporal tumor *(arrows)* that histologically proved to be a glioblastoma multiforme, a rare tumor in children.

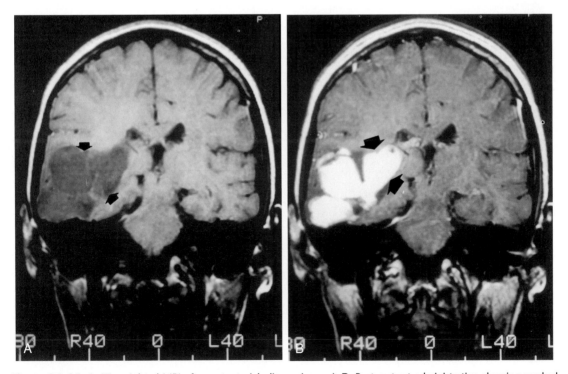

Figure 36–15. A, T1-weighted MRI of supratentorial glioma *(arrows).* **B,** Postcontrast administration showing marked enhancement of the lesion *(arrows).*

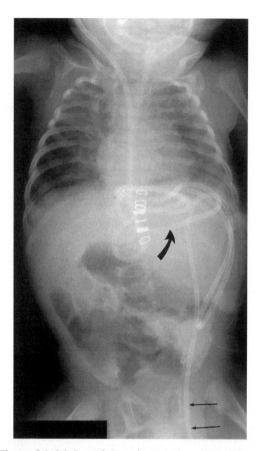

Figure 36–16. Frontal view of ventriculoperitoneal shunt showing the tip heading into the scrotum *(straight arrows)* with resultant shunt malfunction. Extra length of shunt *(curved arrow)* routinely placed in the young child to allow for linear growth of the child.

13) that enhances brightly with contrast. Imaging of the spinal canal is also indicated in these tumors to evaluate the patient for metastases in this region, the so-called drop metastases. This is usually accomplished by MRI, although CT myelography is still used in some institutions.

Brain stem gliomas commonly arise in the pons with diffuse infiltration both caudally and proximally. Hydrocephalus usually occurs, but it is a late finding. Imaging by CT is inferior to MRI because of the bone artifact that occurs when trying to image the brain stem. MRI gives an accurate measurement of the tumor and more easily shows how the lesion affects the adjacent structures. The MRI images usually show symmetrical expansion of the brain stem with compression of adjacent cisterns and the fourth ventricle. The lesion is frequently isointense to hyperintense on T2-weighted images. Enhancement with contrast is variable.

Supratentorial astrocytomas are of variable histologic morphology and appearance on imaging. They may be cystic, solid, or both, and they may or may not have calcification (Fig. 36–14). Contrast enhancement is variable on both CT and MRI. Before contrast is given on MRI, the appearance is also variable on both T1- and T2-weighted images (Fig. 36–15).

MISCELLANEOUS

Patients who have previously been shunted for hydrocephalus can have shunt malfunction that can result in abnormal neurologic signs and symptoms as well as headache. The shunt can break; there can be abnormal absorption of CSF by the peritoneum (so-called CSF pseudocyst), and blockage of the shunt. To evaluate the shunt fully, plain films in both frontal (Fig. 36–16) and lateral views of the entire shunt should be obtained as well as a cranial CT scan to look for ventricular enlargement.

Chapter 37

The Child or Adolescent with a Headache

Children younger than 5 years rarely have a headache without underlying illness. But older children and adolescents frequently have tension and stress headaches and occasional migraines. If they can be sorted out, those patients with real underlying illness are those that need imaging to determine the cause of the headache. Entities discussed in other chapters include the following: intracranial hemorrhage, mass lesions, meningitis, and other intracranial infections. Other entities include sinusitis, mastoiditis, and dental abscess.

DENTAL ABSCESS

A dentist makes the diagnosis of a dental abscess, but it can be screened with a panorex view of the mandible. This view is of the entire mandible and most of the maxilla. The problem with the view is that it is a long exposure and the patient must be able to sit long enough and high enough in the chair for the machine to make an adequate examination. Therefore, most patients less than 5 years old are not capable of having this type of examination performed. Mandible views must then be substituted but are not as diagnostic.

SINUSITIS

Sinusitis is frequently a clinical diagnosis, but when imaging is required, plain films of the sinuses are an adequate starting point. The definitive examination for sinusitis is with an unenhanced CT. Since this examination is more costly than plain films, it is usually reserved for those patients who need the aid of an otolaryngologist. The CT can best view a potential bony abnormality that might interfere with sinus drainage and, therefore, need a surgical procedure to achieve a cure.

Radiographic Findings

The sinuses appear aerated at varying ages. The maxillary and ethmoid sinuses start to aerate at

birth, but they are difficult to see by plain film radiograph until at least 1 year of age. The sphenoid sinus starts its aeration at approximately 3 years of age, and the frontal sinus at around 5 to 6 years of age.

The standard views of the sinuses include the following:

- The Waters view (Fig. 37–1), which is a slightly angled frontal view best for viewing the maxillary sinuses and the anterior ethmoid air cells
- The lateral view, which is best for viewing the sphenoid sinus and lateral view of the

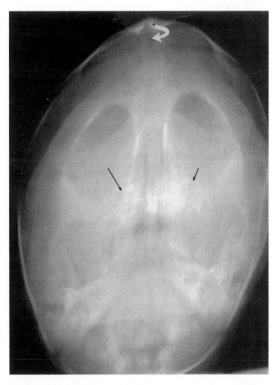

Figure 37–1. Waters view in a neonate. The maxillary sinuses are difficult to see in this infant *(straight arrows)*. It is incidentally noted that the patient has metopic synostosis *(curved arrow)*, which causes the orbits to be closer together than usual (hypoteloric).

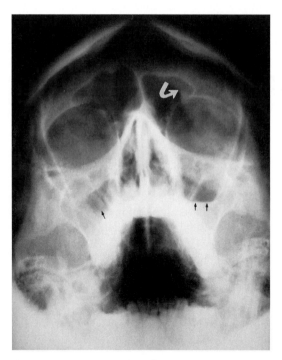

Figure 37–2. Sinusitis with air-fluid levels *(straight arrows)* in the maxillary sinuses as well as mucosal thickening *(curved arrow)*.

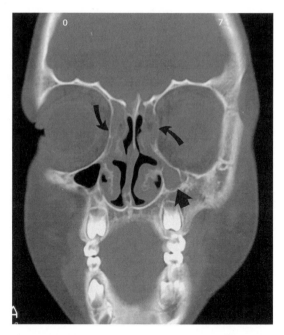

Figure 37–3. Coronal CT scan of abnormal sinuses. The maxillary sinus on the left is totally opaque *(straight arrow)* and the ethmoids are airless, as well *(curved arrows)*.

frontal sinus as well as the soft tissues in the nasopharynx such as the tonsils and adenoids
- The frontal view, which is best for evaluating the frontal sinuses and the posterior ethmoid air cells. The ethmoid air cells, although seen somewhat on plain radiographs, are still better seen with CT scanning.

The plain film findings of acute sinusitis are nonspecific but include air-fluid levels, opacification of a sinus, and mucosal thickening (Fig. 37–2). Chronic sinusitis usually causes mucosal thickening and sometimes polyp formation. Remember: A single opaque sinus, usually maxillary, should be treated with antibiotics and reradiographed in 1 month to make sure that the sinus was not opaque because of a tumor (i.e., rhabdomyosarcoma). Occasionally, plain films are not helpful in making the diagnosis of sinusitis. If imaging is still desired, CT scan can show the abnormality well. Views taken in either the axial or coronal plane are best (Fig. 37–3). Ear, nose, and throat surgeons frequently prefer the direct coronal plane, but this view can be difficult to obtain in a sedated child. Therefore, axial images are usually done in these circumstances and then coronal reconstructed images are obtained on the computer.

MRI examinations are usually not performed for the diagnosis of sinusitis because the MRI can show the mucosal abnormality, but it does not reveal any bony abnormality that might need surgical intervention. In addition, MRI is quite expensive.

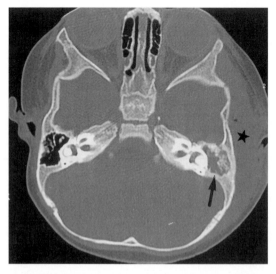

Figure 37–4. Abnormal mastoid air cells *(arrow)* on the left with associated cellulitis *(star)*.

Sometimes, CT and MRI scans are performed for other reasons, and the sinuses are noted to be abnormal. A crying child can have abnormal appearing sinuses, so the clinical correlation as to the presence or absence of sinusitis is crucial for accurate diagnosis.

MASTOIDITIS

Mastoiditis can also present with headache. The best plain radiographic view for visualization of the mastoid air cells is the Towne view, which emphasizes the posterior aspect of the skull. However, plain film diagnosis is inaccurate since the mastoids may have aerated differently and, therefore, simulate disease when it is not really present. CT can evaluate possible bony destruction and ossicular displacement (Fig. 37–4). MRI can be used to diagnose intracranial spread, if present. On unenhanced MRI scans, abnormal hyperintense signal is seen on T2-weighted images.

Index

Note: Page numbers followed by f refer to figures; page numbers followed by t refer to tables.